Boosting Brain Health with Supplements: Top Choices for Cognitive Support

A Comprehensive Guide to Nutrients, Supplements, and Lifestyle Choices for Optimal Brain Health

Nena Buenaventura

Copyright

Disclaimer Statement

The information presented in "**Boosting Brain Health with Supplements: Top Choices for Cognitive Support**" is intended solely for educational and informational purposes. This book does not replace professional medical advice, diagnosis, or treatment. Always seek the guidance of a qualified healthcare provider with any questions regarding medical conditions or treatments, including those related to cognitive health and the use of supplements. The opinions and experiences shared here reflect the research and understanding of the author and are not necessarily universally applicable or endorsed by medical professionals.

Consult a physician or licensed healthcare provider before starting any new supplement regimen, dietary changes, exercise program, or other health-related activities. Certain supplements, especially when combined with medications or existing health conditions, can have adverse effects. Individual responses to dietary and lifestyle changes, supplements, and health practices will vary. Although efforts have been made to ensure accuracy, the author and publisher disclaim any liability for risks or damages, directly or indirectly, resulting from the use or application of the contents within this book.

The personal stories and testimonials shared in this document are individual experiences and may not reflect the typical results of using supplements.

This document is not a substitute for professional medical advice.

Table of Contents

Preface

In today's fast-paced, information-rich world, our brains are constantly challenged to keep up. We rely on mental clarity, focus, memory, and resilience to excel in our personal and professional lives, yet many of us face increasing cognitive demands that can leave us feeling fatigued, stressed, or mentally strained. Meanwhile, a growing awareness of cognitive decline and conditions such as Alzheimer's disease has sparked a search for ways to support brain health proactively. This book, Boosting Brain Health with Supplements: Top Choices for Cognitive Support, is a response to that need—a resource to help you navigate the journey of maintaining and enhancing cognitive well-being.

This book combines practical knowledge, scientific insights, and actionable advice on using supplements to support brain function at every stage of life. We'll explore the key vitamins, minerals, and herbal allies that offer natural support for memory, concentration, stress management, and overall mental energy. Alongside these supplements, we'll discuss the essential role of lifestyle choices, such as nutrition, exercise, sleep, and mindfulness, and how these daily habits powerfully reinforce cognitive health.

Supplementation, however, is just one piece of the puzzle. It's equally important to understand how to incorporate supplements effectively and safely. This book will guide you in selecting high-quality products, evaluating supplement claims, and making informed decisions based on research. And because each person's cognitive journey is unique, we'll share real-life stories from students, professionals, and everyday individuals who have found success through the mindful integration of cognitive health practices.

Boosting Brain Health with Supplements is more than a guide to brain health; it's an invitation to embrace a lifelong path of cognitive wellness. By helping you craft a personalized plan, set achievable goals, and navigate potential setbacks, this book aims to empower you to take control of your brain health. Whether you're just starting or looking to deepen your practice, I hope this resource becomes a companion on your journey to a more vibrant, resilient mind.

Welcome to a future of cognitive vitality and sustained mental well-being.

Awakening the Mind

The Journey Begins

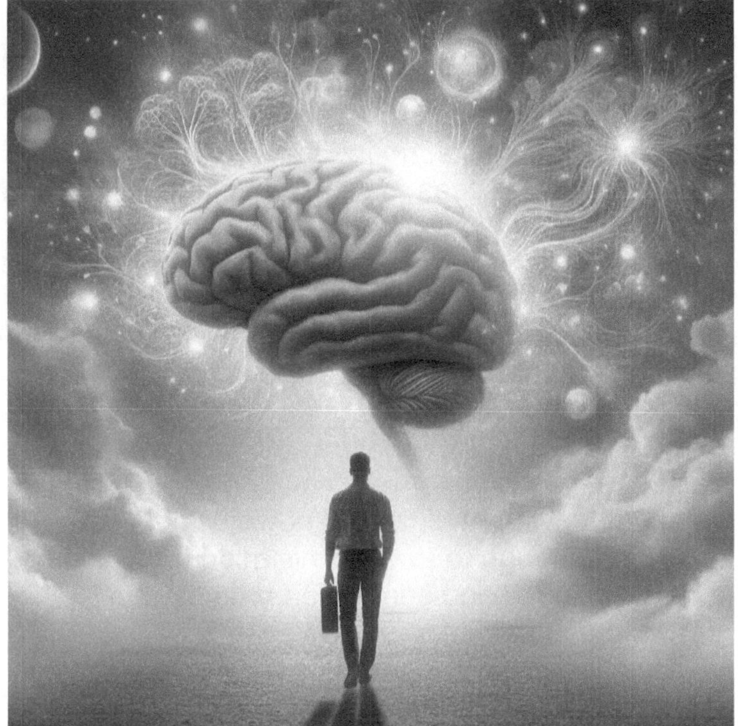

Sam stood at the crossroads of his life, burdened by an overwhelming sense of fatigue and mental fog that had slowly seeped into his daily existence. With every passing day, he felt his cognitive sharpness fading, replaced by frustration and a gnawing question: How could he reclaim his focus and clarity? The weight of stacks of unfinished tasks loomed heavily over him, each uncompleted item a testament to his dwindling motivation.

As he sifted through countless articles online, the promise of cognitive supplements began to shine like a beacon of hope. Words such as natural, enhanced performance, and mind clarity stirred a flicker of excitement within him. Yet, skepticism clung to the edges of his thoughts. Would these supplements actually deliver results, or were they merely another marketing ploy? Regardless, the desperation to escape this mental quagmire pushed him toward action.

With a list in hand and a heart full of determination, Sam made his way to the local health store, yet doubt lingered. Standing in the aisle surrounded by colorful bottles and bold claims, he felt the enormity of his decision. What if he was making a mistake? What if he wasted money, time, and hope? Just as he turned to leave, a whisper of resolve took hold. This journey was about more than just supplements; it was about reclaiming a part of himself he thought he'd lost forever. Each supplement he carefully selected represented a step toward empowerment, but as the door swung closed behind him, Sam realized the journey was just beginning. Filled with both anticipation and unease, he now faced the weight of the unknown: Would these changes be enough to awaken his mind, or would he one day look back and see a road not yet traveled, regrets clinging to his footsteps?

Understanding Cognitive Health

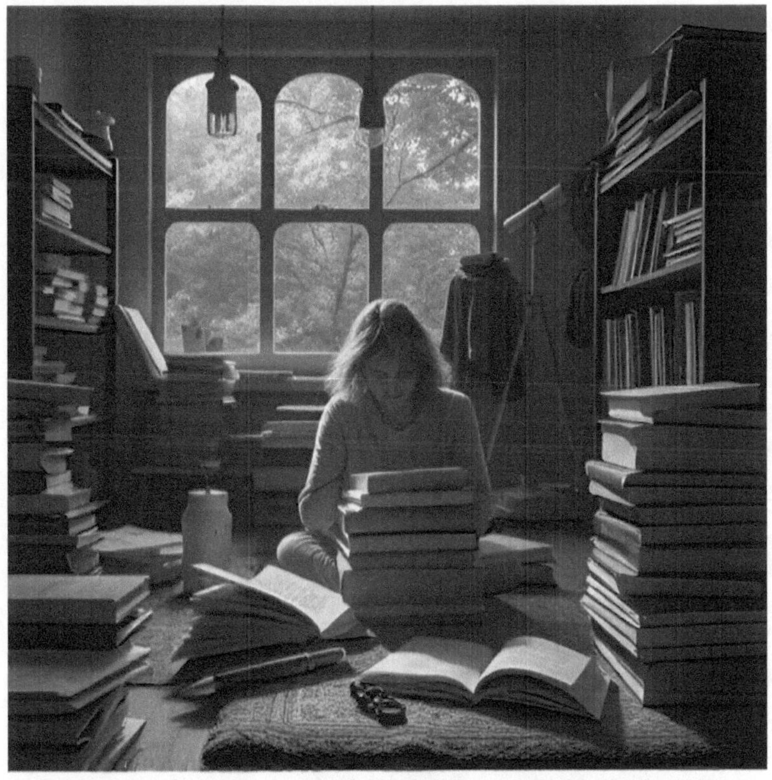

Sarah sat in the dim light of her cramped study, surrounded by stacks of textbooks and notes. The pressure of her academic responsibilities weighed heavily on her shoulders. Each day felt like a relentless cycle of lectures, assignments, and late-night cramming. Yet, an unsettling thought loomed at the back of her mind: was she truly equipped to succeed in this demanding environment? Determined to find answers, Sarah delved into research that promised insights into cognitive health, hoping to unlock potential pathways to academic success.

As she embarked on this journey, Sarah discovered that cognitive health was a multifaceted realm, rooted in various pillars: nutrition, exercise, sleep, and mindfulness. Each component played a crucial role in shaping not only a person's mental clarity and memory but also their overall emotional well-being. The deeper she dug, the more it became clear; she was not merely a student, but an architect of her own cognitive landscape. However, just as she began to piece together her plan, doubts crept in—could mere changes in lifestyle truly elevate her performance? Could she really alter the course of her studies through these adjustments?

With a newfound sense of urgency, Sarah meticulously crafted a list of goals aimed at enhancing her cognitive health. She introduced vibrant fruits and vegetables into her meals, incorporated brisk walks into her daily routine, and established a strict sleep schedule. Each positive change seemed to ripple through her mind and body, reawakening a sense of potential. Yet, in the quiet moments, the weight of her academic pressures loomed larger than ever. Would these efforts be enough to secure the future she desired? Time was slipping away, and the stakes were higher than she could have ever imagined. In the shadows of her study, an unsettling truth emerged: while knowledge was power, the battle for cognitive health was just beginning.

The Role of Supplements

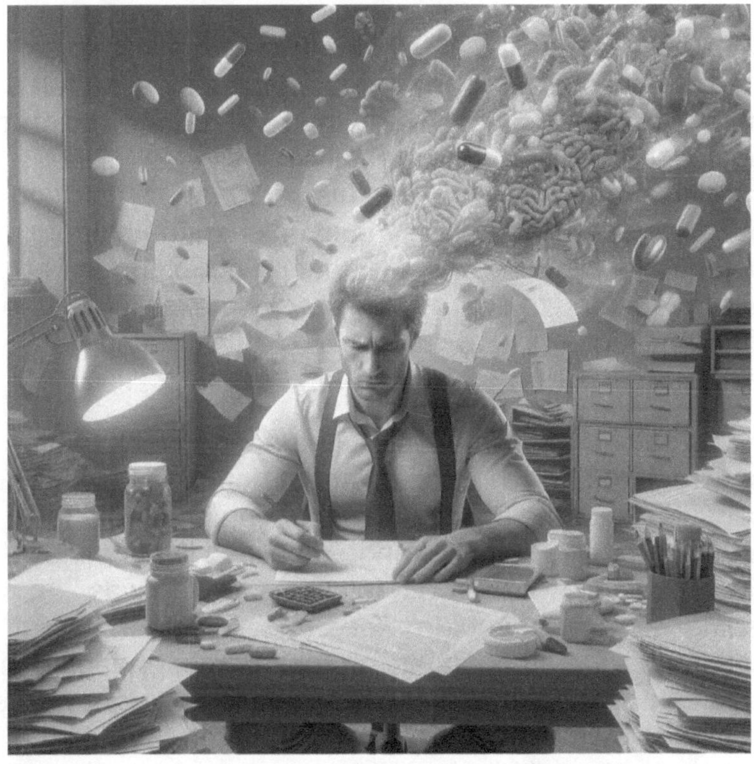

Mike sat at his cluttered desk, papers strewn about like the thoughts swirling in his head. He had always been a hard worker, but lately, the demands of his job felt insurmountable. He had heard whispers around the office about coworkers boosting their productivity with supplements, and the curiosity began to gnaw at him. What if these tiny capsules held the key to unlocking a sharper, more efficient version of himself?

With a determined mindset, he began his investigation. Hours turned into days as he researched the various supplements touted for cognitive enhancement. Omega-3 fatty acids promised to improve memory and mood. Ginkgo biloba was said to sharpen focus. The choices were overwhelming, yet he felt an excitement bubbling within him. This was no longer just about improving his work performance; it was about reclaiming his mental clarity and fortitude.

Mike decided to take action, starting with a visit to a local health store. As he navigated the aisles, he felt a rush of hope. The walls were lined with brightly colored bottles, each one a potential ally in his quest for cognitive resilience. He filled his cart carefully, picking out adaptations he hoped would unleash the hidden potential of his mind. Yet, a lingering doubt tugged at him. Would these supplements really make a difference, or was it all just a placebo, a fleeting fantasy?

As he settled back into his routine after a week of his new regimen, the initial excitement began to wane. The capsules became a part of his morning ritual, but the urgency for noticeable change amplified in his mind. Each passing hour at work felt like a test he was failing—a race he couldn't keep up with. Other colleagues were constantly on their game, engaging in fluid conversations while he grasped for the right words, confused by the noise of his own thoughts. Would the supplements pull him from this mire, or was he destined to wallow forever in the shadows of his potential?

Frustration mounted as Mike clutched his head, the stress creeping ever deeper into his quiet moments. He poured over reviews and studies, convinced that he was missing some secret logic to making the desired leap. The contrast between those who thrived and himself weighed heavy on his shoulders. Every conflicting piece of advice he encountered only served to deepen his doubt.

Just as desperation started to carve itself a seat at his table, an unexpected email pinged into his inbox. It was an invitation to a workshop on cognitive health and supplements, hosted by a renowned expert. The possibility of personal guidance ignited a flicker of hope within him. But would this be the breakthrough he desperately sought, or yet another path leading to disappointment?

With mixed emotions, Mike registered for the workshop, feeling both anticipation and fear. As the event approached, he understood one thing: he needed to confront his doubts head-on. This could either be the final push towards the cognitive freedom he craved or a reminder of the barriers he'd built around himself. The stakes were high, and it wouldn't just be Mike's mind on the line—it would determine the trajectory of his career and how he perceived his worth.

The Power of Nutrients

Vitamins for the Brain

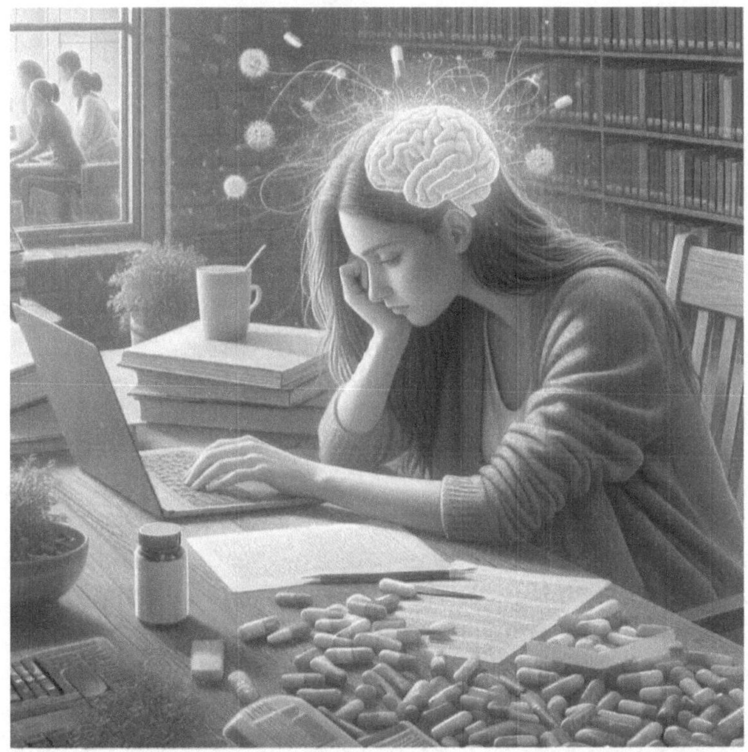

Amidst the clattering of keyboards and faint chatter in the library, Julia felt the weight of her responsibilities pressing down like an iron cloak. Juggling her coursework, part-time job, and social life left her mentally drained, an echo of worry brushing against the edges of her thoughts. The late-night studying was no longer effective, and the vibrant energy she once had was replaced with a dull fatigue she couldn't shake off.

Determined to reclaim her focus and vitality, she dove into research about vitamins that could potentially turn the tide. The pages spoke of B vitamins, complex yet essential allies in enhancing cognitive function, energy, and mood. Thiamine, riboflavin, and niacin each played a vital role like instruments in a symphony, and Julia felt a flicker of hope that perhaps these nutrients could compose a solution to her struggles.

With newfound determination, Julia mapped out a plan. She organized her meals, incorporating more leafy greens, eggs, and legumes, each a storehouse of vitamins essential for her brain. However, as she reached for a multivitamin supplement to bridge any gaps, uncertainty seeped in. Would this be enough to awaken the dormant capacity within her mind? The more she dug, the more questions surfaced, creating a storm of unease as she reflected upon her recent performance and the crumbling expectations she had set for herself.

As the sun dipped below the horizon, casting shadows across the office, David leaned back in his chair, rubbing his temples in frustration. The deadlines loomed closer, but his concentration was slipping through his fingers like grains of sand. He had heard whispers of minerals playing a pivotal role in cognitive function, but the deeper he explored, the more he realized how crucial they were to his daily performance.

Magnesium and zinc danced into his awareness, each promising to combat fatigue and enhance memory recall. Excited yet skeptical, David started to incorporate nuts and seeds into his afternoon routine, convinced that a dietary shift could ultimately propel him through the thickets of fatigue. Each bite felt like a small victory, but the nagging doubt lingered: Was he doing enough? Could these changes truly fortify him against the mental fatigue that seeped in like an unwelcome cold?

The stakes rose as the final meeting of the week edged closer, and as David turned to his supplements, he felt the tension building—a crescendo of anticipation mixed with anxiety. Would he crack under pressure or rise to the challenge, fortified by his newfound knowledge of minerals? The clock ticked down relentlessly, and with each passing second, the burden of expectation weighed heavier on his shoulders.

Emma stared at her computer screen, heart racing, as the words blurred before her eyes. The hours spent scouring through research felt futile; her mind was clouded, engulfed in a haze that left her struggling to find clarity. It was then that she stumbled upon antioxidants—powerful compounds that could potentially reduce oxidative stress and improve cognitive function.

Fascinated, she learned about vitamins C and E, not just as immune boosters but as protective forces against the mental fog that had settled in. She envisioned a vibrant rainbow of fruits and vegetables decorating her plate, each morsel bursting with the promise of clearer thinking and renewed energy. But as excitement flickered in her chest, a darker thought threatened to overshadow her enthusiasm: what if adding these foods and supplements didn't yield the results she so desperately craved?

The upcoming exam loomed like a storm cloud, anxiety crackling through the air around her. It was a test not just of her knowledge, but of her ability to adapt and overcome obstacles. Would the antioxidants be her safeguard, or simply another mirage in her quest for success? With the clock ticking down, Emma steeled herself, the weight of doubt mixing with a fierce desire to climb the mountain that was her impending test.

Minerals That Matter

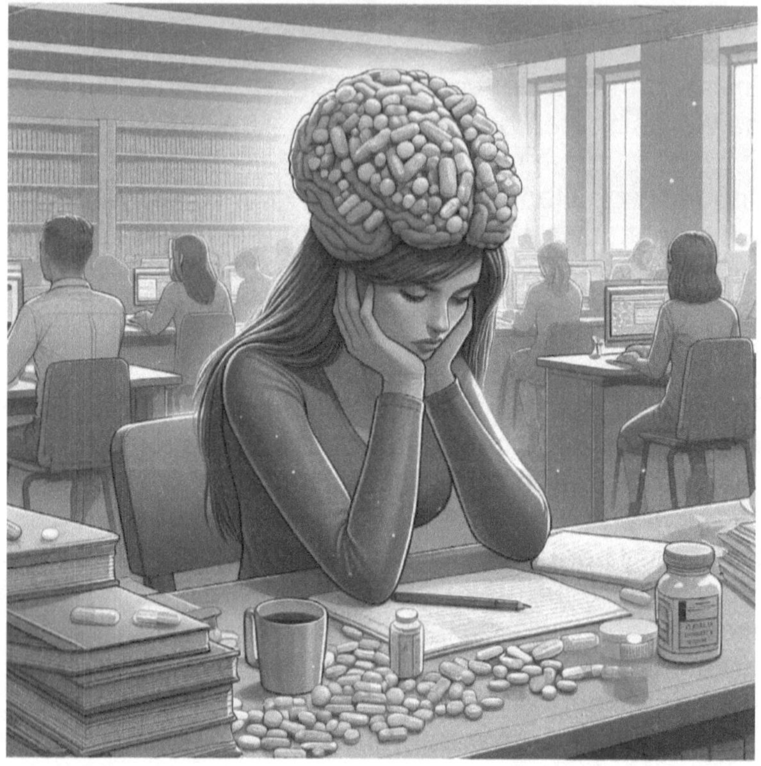

David felt the weight of exhaustion creeping in as he stared at his computer screen, with tasks piling up like an unyielding mountain before him. Each hour dragged on longer than the last, and with that, his focus began to flicker. He had heard whispers of how certain minerals can boost cognitive function, but he never took it seriously—until now. The clear realization that his mind was faltering pushed him to dive deeper into the world of nutritional science.

He started his research with Magnesium, a mineral often overlooked. Known as a powerful brain booster, magnesium was linked to improved memory and cognitive stability. He discovered how it plays a vital role in the synaptic function within the brain and how a deficiency could lead to anxiety and memory issues.

David's eyebrows knitted together as he read about its potential benefits, igniting a flicker of hope: could this be the key to unlocking his mental clarity?

His exploration continued into Zinc, a mineral he knew little about but had often been mentioned in the same breath as cognitive health. As he read studies highlighting zinc's importance in stabilizing neural structures and its role in regulating neurotransmitters, David felt a growing urgency. Time slipped away, his responsibilities loomed larger, and with every passing minute, he felt increasingly desperate to reclaim his focus. The stakes were high; he couldn't afford to falter in his responsibilities—a promotion hung in the balance, demanding every ounce of his mental acumen. David's breath quickened as he poured over the information, the weight of what was to come pressing down on him.

The rhythm of his anxious heartbeat pulsed in his ears as he learned about Iron, another mineral crucial for cognitive performance. Suddenly, a picture formed in his mind: the blood flowing with energy, carrying oxygen necessary for his brain to function at its peak. It sent a jolt of anxiety right to his core—was he truly nourishing himself, or had the daily grind begun to erode his mental well-being? The terror of stagnation and the uncertainty of his capacity flooded his thoughts, leaving him writhing in self-doubt.

Feeling overwhelmed, he took a moment to breathe. But then there it was, nestled among all this newfound knowledge: the creeping realization that change was necessary but fraught with its own challenges. Would he take the plunge into fortifying his mind with minerals? Or would the fear of failing at yet another attempt hold him back? With the clock ticking and deadlines approaching, David found himself standing at a precipice. One decision could lead him to mastery of his mind—or further into the abyss of distraction and collapse. The tension coiled tighter within him, as he prepared to choose what path he would take amidst this whirlwind of pressure.

Understanding Antioxidants

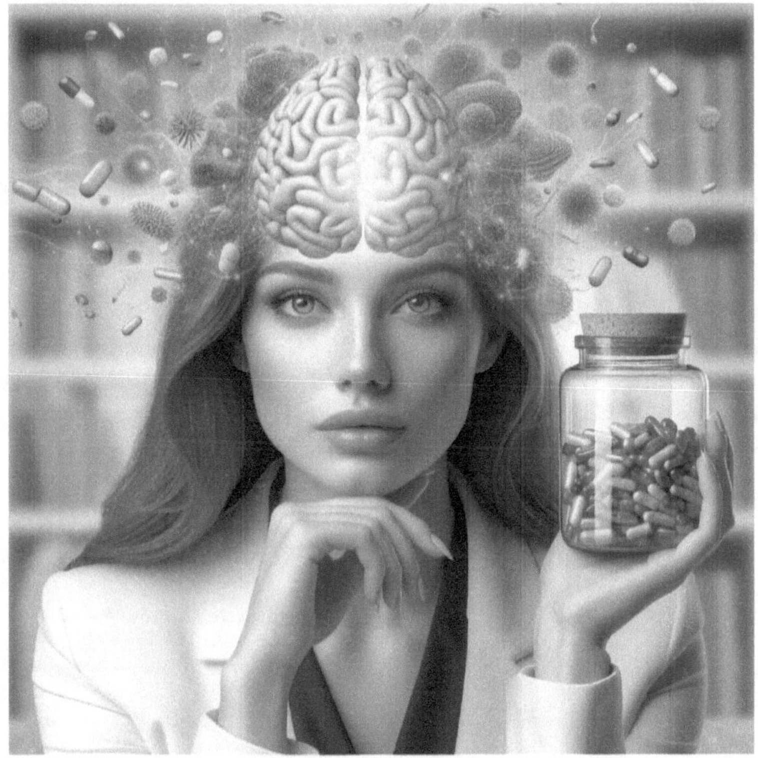

As Emma delved deeper into her quest for mental clarity, she stumbled upon the fascinating world of antioxidants. Initially, she thought of them only in the context of physical health, but her recent readings highlighted their crucial role in cognitive function as well. With classes piling up, managing her time had never felt more overwhelming. She needed a way to enhance her focus, and the promise of antioxidants quickly caught her attention.

Through a series of articles and studies, she learned that oxidative stress could damage brain cells over time, leading to cognitive decline—a looming threat to her academic performance. Determined to arm herself with knowledge, Emma began researching foods rich in antioxidants, like berries, nuts, and dark chocolate. The thought of including these vibrant foods in her diet brought a new wave of excitement into her routine, but she wondered if merely eating these foods would be enough to combat the relentless stress of her studies.

Days turned into weeks, and Emma noticed subtle changes in her concentration levels. But as midterms approached, she found herself caught in a whirlwind of anxiety and sleepless nights. The more she tried to harness the power of antioxidants, the more elusive her focus became. Just when she thought she was on top of things, the pressure mounted, casting a shadow over her progress. It wasn't just about the food anymore; she realized she needed a concrete strategy to complement her newfound knowledge, but doubt crept in as the stakes rose higher.

Finding Balance

Nutrition vs. Supplements

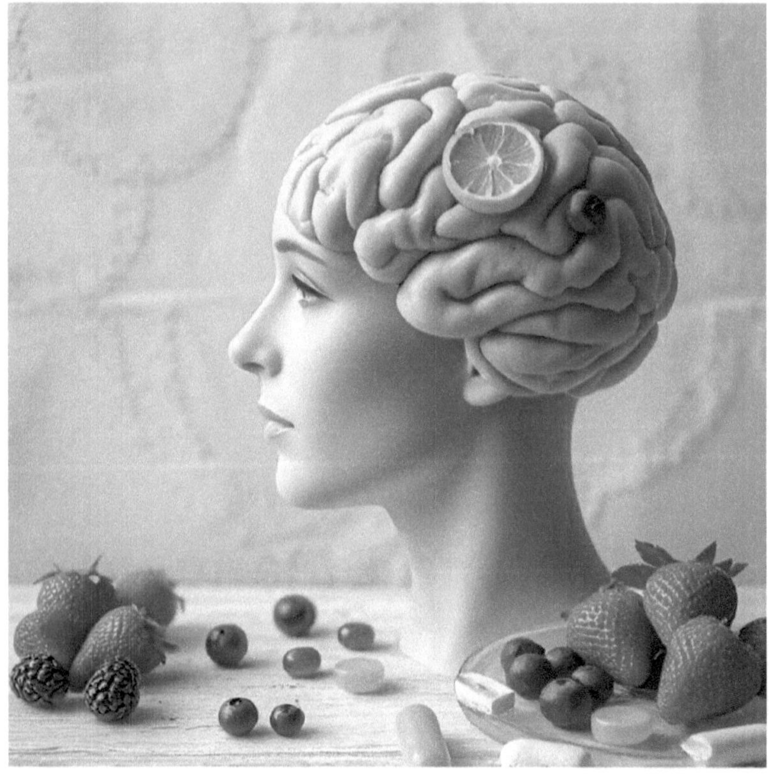

Chris stood in the grocery aisle, a kaleidoscope of colors surrounding him as he perused the fresh fruits and vegetables. Just a week prior, he had been engrossed in an online debate that would set the tone for his evolving perspective on nutrition and supplements. On one side were advocates for a whole foods approach, embellishing the virtues of nutritious meals crafted from scratch. On the opposing end, the convenience and targeted benefits of supplements called to him—tiny capsules promising enhanced focus, mental clarity, and energy. With every passing moment in the aisle, Chris felt the burden of choice weigh heavier on his shoulders.

His mind flicked back to a conversation with his colleague, Melissa, who passionately argued that nothing could replace the complete array of nutrients found in whole foods. "Supplements are just that," she had said, her voice echoing in his memory, "Supplements. They can't compete with the richness of natural food sources." Yet, as Chris studied the intricate labels on energy-boosting supplements, he acknowledged the merit behind her words. Was it really wise to rely on pills to fill the gaps left by a busy lifestyle that pulled him away from cooking fresh meals? The tension between the two worlds left him feeling uncertain.

After spending an hour wrestling with the options, Chris finally closed his eyes, inhaling deeply to ground himself. The aroma of ripening produce mingled in the air—a bouquet of potential and nourishment. He envisioned a meticulously planned day filled with nutrient-rich meals, only to have it overshadowed by the reality of time constraints and fatigue. Balancing the delights of cooking and eating well with the allure of the supplement aisle was turning out to be more complex than he had anticipated. Would he ever find a harmonious rhythm that embraced both sides, or was he destined to be consumed by the struggle of choices forever? The answer loomed like a dark cloud, and Chris felt a sense of urgency to resolve the tension brewing in his mind.

Creating a Dietary Plan

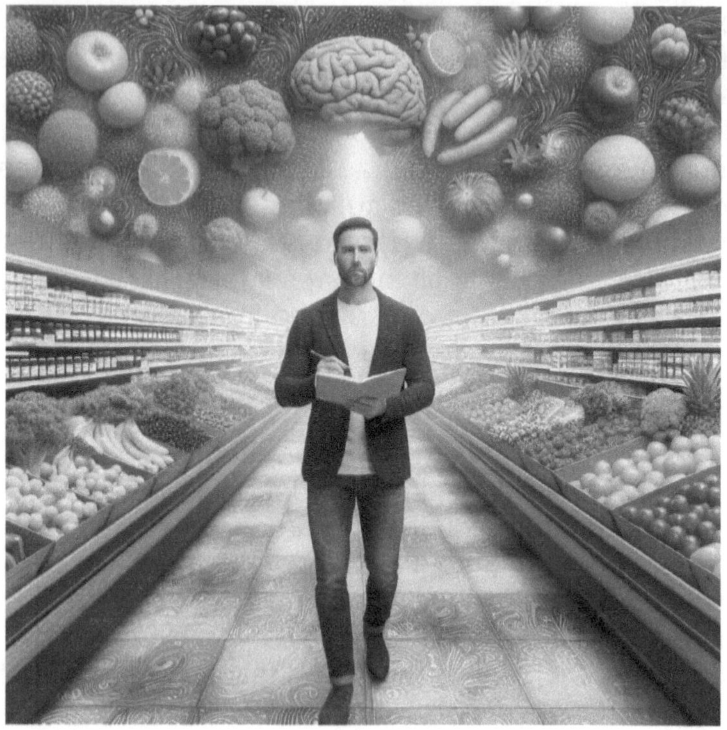

As Alex sat at his kitchen table, a whirlwind of thoughts danced through his mind. The desire to improve his cognitive abilities weighed heavily on him, compelling him to put pen to paper. His friends had always told him that nutrition was key to optimal brain function, but now, it felt critical. Each word that flowed from his pencil was a step toward the clarity and focus he so desperately needed.

He carefully jotted down notes on various foods known to enhance cognitive performance: fatty fish rich in Omega-3s, leafy greens loaded with antioxidants, and nuts bursting with healthy fats. The colors of the foods swirled in his imagination, painting a vibrant picture of a balanced diet that could bolster not only his mind but also his spirit.

However, doubt crept in as he reflected on his busy lifestyle. Could he really pull this off amidst his tight schedule? The images of frozen meals and caffeine-laden snacks flashed in his mind, taunting him with the reality of convenience over nutrition. Yet, as he stared at the blank page, he felt that this was a crucial turning point. The stakes were higher than ever; this commitment could change everything.

Inspired, he started visualizing his days ahead. Breakfasts filled with yogurt and berries, quick lunch wraps brimming with spinach and salmon, snacks of almonds and dark chocolate hidden in his bag. Motivation surged through him like a jolt of electricity as he merged practicality with ambition. But just as he began feeling confident, an ominous thought flickered in his mind: What if he stumbled? What if the challenges derailed him before he even started?

Determined, he pushed such negativity aside, but tension gripped his heart. What if he failed to adhere to his plan? The fear of slipping back into his old habits loomed large, a specter haunting his aspirations. He envisioned the mounting pressures of exams and deadlines looming on the horizon, creating a storm of uncertainty. Would his dietary changes hold strong against the chaos of his life?

With each stroke of his pen, he penned affirmations of resilience and commitment at the bottom of the page. Yet, deep within, a flicker of anxiety remained. The thought of creating this dietary plan was merely the beginning—what lay beyond it was an equally daunting journey of consistency and discipline. Alex glanced around his kitchen, the weight of the moment settling in as he recognized the enormity of the challenge ahead. Could he truly strike a balance that eluded him for so long?

The Importance of Hydration

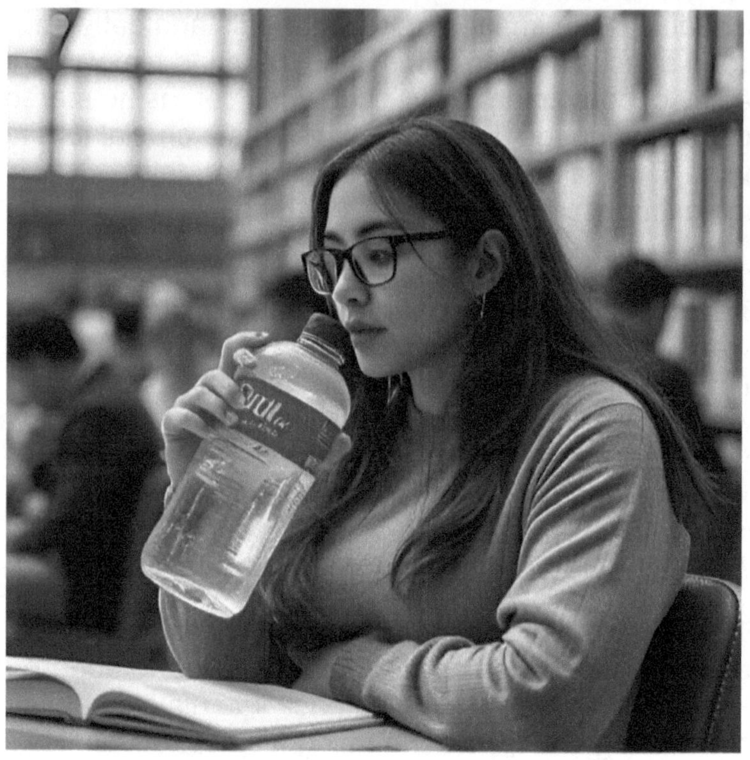

Tina sat in the crowded library, her mind swirling with equations and concepts that seemed to float just beyond her grasp. She had read the textbook, attended every lecture, and diligently reviewed her notes, yet a nagging fatigue threatened to pull her focus away from the pages. It wasn't until a friend casually mentioned how dehydration could affect cognitive function that a thought sparked in her mind. Had she been drinking enough water?

The idea lingered as she sipped from her nearly empty water bottle, the familiar plastic crinkling in her hand. Every sip felt like a small victory, yet she couldn't shake the feeling that she was falling behind. With exams looming, the pressure mounted, and she instinctively reached for yet another energy drink. The jitteriness in her fingers intensified, but so did the confusion swirling in her mind. Could she really afford to ignore something as simple as hydration?

As she stared out the window, observing the world outside bustling with life, a realization struck. Hydration wasn't just about drinking water; it symbolized the support she needed in her quest for academic success. It was about taking care of herself holistically, acknowledging that every element of her well-being intertwined. With renewed resolve, she stood up, the decision crystallizing in her mind—I need to take my hydration seriously. It's time to reclaim the focus I've lost before it's too late.

Determined to turn her anxiety into proactive habits, Tina made her way to the campus café. As she filled her water bottle to the brim, she felt waves of empowerment washing over her. Still, as she left the café, a fleeting shadow of doubt curled in the back of her mind. Would drinking more water really make a difference? The weight of her upcoming exams pressed down, and she couldn't help but wonder if she was flexing her mental muscles the right way. Shaking her head, she banished the thought; she had made the choice to prioritize her health, and that alone was a step towards balance.

The Essential
Supplements

Omega-3 Fatty Acids: The Brain's Best Friend

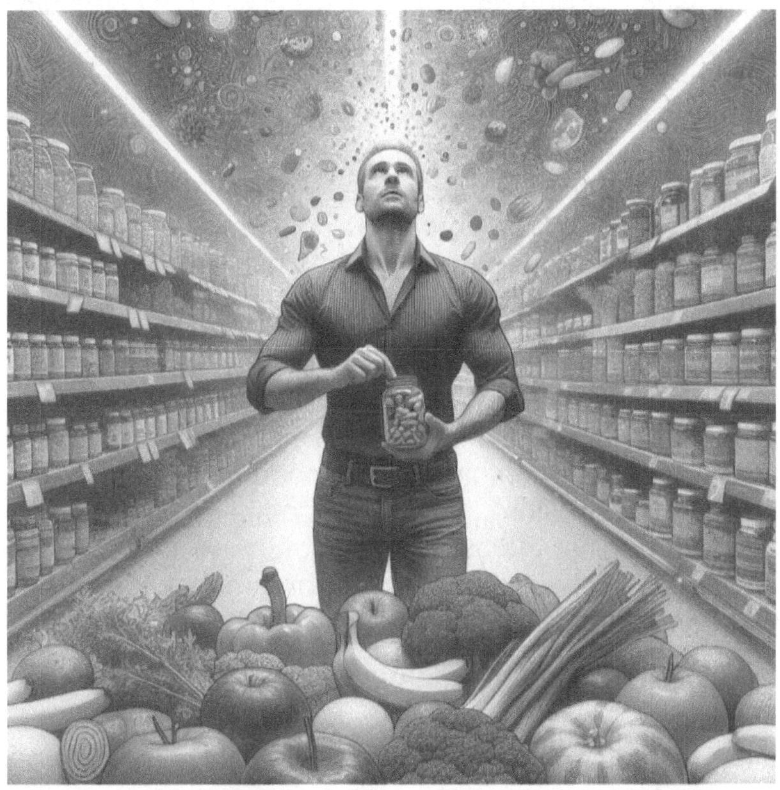

Max sat at his kitchen table, a stack of books about cognitive health spread out in front of him. The morning sun illuminated the pages, casting a warm glow over the dense text that spoke of brain health, memory, and emotional wellbeing. Yet, amidst his quest for knowledge, he felt a growing sense of restlessness, as if something crucial was just beyond his reach.

He had always been curious about Omega-3s, the supposed miracle fats touted as the brain's best friends. As he flipped through the pages, the benefits unfurled like vibrant petals, revealing connections to improved memory and mood stabilization. But could they be the key to unlocking his full potential? There was an urgency in his heart, a feeling that his mental agility was slipping, and he needed to act swiftly.

With each passing day, he noticed the fog of distraction creeping in, making it harder to concentrate on his studies and engage in conversations. Friends had begun to voice their concerns, noting his frequent forgetfulness and unwarranted irritability. That evening, as he sipped a smoothie packed with leafy greens and fruits, the thought of Omega-3s consumed him. He had to find a way to integrate them into his life.

Max's exploration led him to fish oil supplements, capsules shimmering in their pristine packaging, offering promises of cognitive enhancement. Yet, doubt nagged at him; would they actually help him? In a moment of determination, he reached for the bottle at his local health store, his fingers trembling as they brushed against the cool surface of the container. He could feel the weight of his decision pressing down on him, heightened by his longing for clarity and focus.

That night, as he lay in bed staring at the ceiling, uncertainty and hope twined together. He envisioned the impact Omega-3s could have on his life, fuelling his passion for learning. Yet another part of him feared the prospect of disappointment. What if he poured his heart into this, only to find it was yet another remedy that promised more than it could deliver? It was a gamble, but he knew he had to try. Morning would come, and with it, his first step toward reclamation.

As Max drifted into a restless sleep, filled with dreams of sharp intellect and emotional balance, a single thought echoed in his mind: Would Omega-3s really prove to be the catalyst for change he desperately sought, or were they just another mirage in the vast desert of cognitive enhancement? The stakes were high, and it felt as if the answers were just around the corner—waiting to unveil themselves in the early dawn light.

B Vitamins: Energy for the Mind

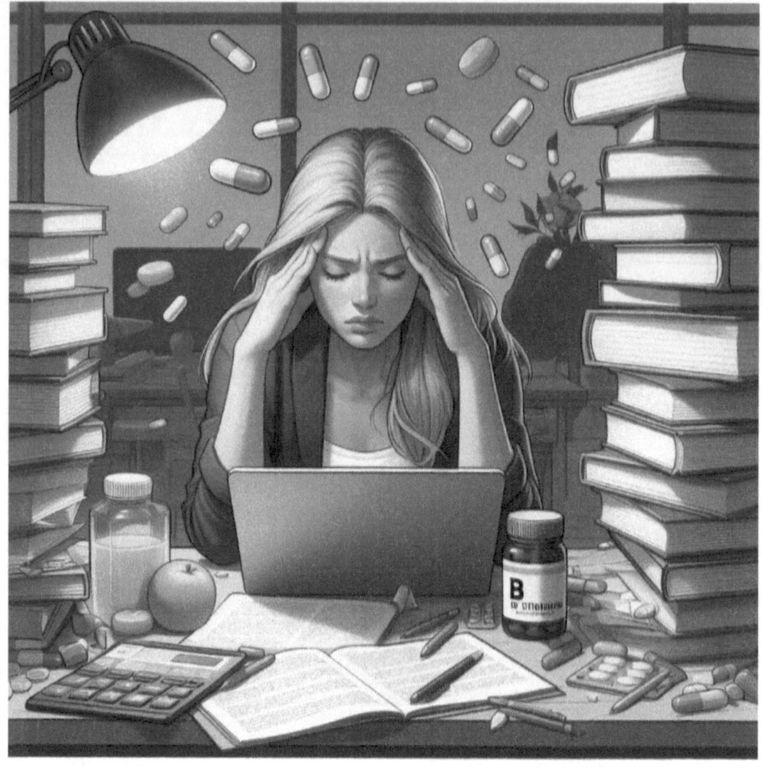

Lily had always struggled with the late-night studying that left her drained and foggy. With exams approaching, she felt the pressure mounting, overwhelming her with anxiety. As she sat at her desk, surrounded by a mountain of textbooks, the questions of how to keep her energy levels from plummeting echoed in her mind. She knew she needed more than just willpower to pull through this stressful time – she needed a plan.

Flipping through the pages of her nutrition book, she stumbled upon a section dedicated to B vitamins. Intrigued, she learned that these essential nutrients played a critical role in brain health and energy production. B1, B2, B3, and particularly B12 caught her attention; they didn't just support physical energy but were vital for cognitive function. Her curiosity turned into determination as she noted the impact these vitamins could have on her study sessions.

With a newfound sense of purpose, Lily ventured to the local health store. She examined bottle after bottle, absorbing information about each supplement. As she stood there, she felt the weight of the decision heavy on her shoulders. What if she invested in these vitamins and saw no change? The self-doubt nagged at her. But deep down, she knew she needed to try something. With a few chosen bottles in her basket, she headed home, excitement and apprehension vying for dominance in her heart.

As the days wore on, the effects of the B vitamins began to reveal themselves. The fog began to lift, replaced by a clarity she hadn't experienced in years. Each study session became more focused, and the moments of panic started to fade. Yet, just when she felt she was catching her breath, a troubling thought crept back in: would her reliance on these supplements become a crutch? Was she truly learning, or merely floating along on a chemical boost? The tension built within her, wrestling with every little victory against the doubt that clouded her mind.

On the eve of her exam, Lily felt a storm brewing inside her. The stakes were higher than ever, and the pressure threatened to crack her newfound confidence. She paced her room, repeating her notes under her breath while wrestling with her unease. The B vitamins had helped, but what if they weren't enough? The night stretched on, each tick of the clock echoing her worries. As she finally settled into bed, exhaustion wrapped around her like a heavy blanket, but sleep eluded her. Tomorrow could change everything, and the profound uncertainty loomed like a shadow over her.

Ginkgo Biloba: Enhancing Memory

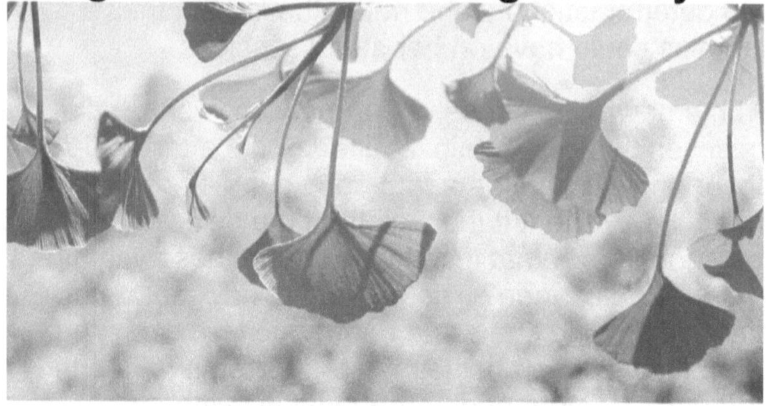

Jacob felt an unshakeable weight on his shoulders as the semester rolled into its final stretch. His notes, scribbled on scattered sheets, were a chaotic representation of his thoughts—jumbled, lost, and fading away like smoke in a breeze. Struggling to keep pace with his classmates, he wandered into the library one afternoon, not for the usual textbooks, but seeking something that could light the fog clouding his mind.

As he browsed the stacks, a colorful brochure caught his eye: Unlock Your Memory Potential with Ginkgo Biloba! It piqued his interest. The world outside buzzed with distractions, yet here, in this quiet haven, the ancient tree known for its remarkable resilience garnered attention for its promises of clarity, focus, and cognitive enhancement. Could this be the answer to his mounting academic pressures?

Jacob delved into the pamphlet, absorbing the enticing claims. Ginkgo Biloba had roots traced back thousands of years in traditional medicine, and modern studies hinted at its effectiveness in boosting memory and sharpened focus. It was whispered to increase blood flow to the brain—could it truly cut through his mental fog and forge a path to success?

Feeling a flicker of hope, Jacob decided to give it a try. He visited the local health store, the soft chime of the bell above the door announcing his arrival into a realm bursting with promise. After a brief conversation with the store clerk, he walked out with a bottle of Ginkgo Biloba, cradled in his palm like a talisman against mediocrity.

Days turned into weeks, and Jacob diligently incorporated the supplement into his routine, nagging disbelief wrestled with burgeoning optimism. But as midterms approached, the pressure morphed into a pit in his stomach. He commenced intensive study sessions, but with each passing hour, anxiety gnawed at him. What if the Ginkgo didn't work? What if he was chasing an illusion?

Late one night, panic began to crack the surface of his resolve. He was two days away from his first test, and as he sat surrounded by notes, the words blurred together, refusing to be absorbed. The sense of having gambled on Ginkgo spiraled into doubt. His hands trembled as he reached for his phone, contemplating a frantic message to a friend, but his fingers hovered hesitantly above the screen.

Then came a breakthrough—or was it a mirage? As he revisited the same passage for the umpteenth time, a spark ignited within him. A fragment of information coalesced, and clarity flickered like a candle caught in the wind. He leaned forward, eyes widening. Could it be? Was the fog beginning to lift? Adrenaline surged through him, pushing back against the tide of despair.

Yet, the question lingered: had Ginkgo truly shifted something within him, or was it merely the fervor of desperation? Tension coiled tightly in his chest as he prepared for the test, oscillating between hope and uncertainty. He knew that the real test would soon reveal itself, but would he shine or falter?

Herbal Allies

Rhodiola Rosea: Stress Support

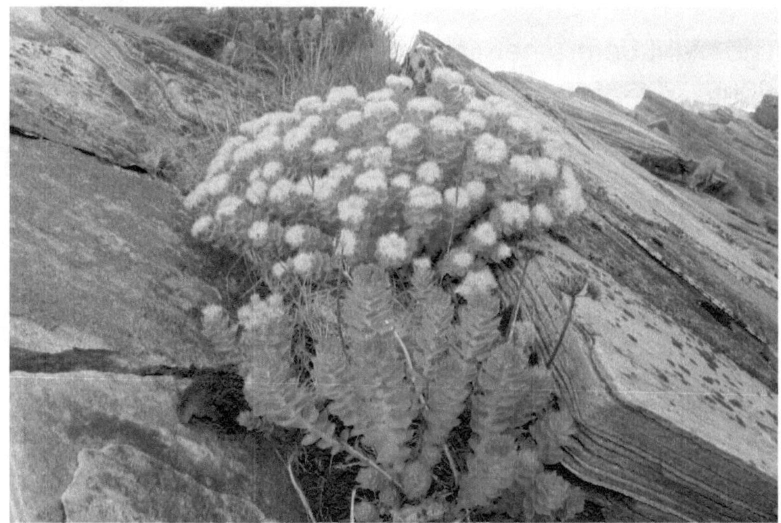

Natalie had always prided herself on her resilience. But as exams approached, she found herself buried under an avalanche of coursework and mounting pressure. Each passing day brought fresh assignments and relentless reminders of what was at stake. The weight of expectation sat heavy on her shoulders, suffocating her once vibrant spirit.

Desperate for relief, Natalie stumbled upon the ancient herb, Rhodiola Rosea, known for its potential to combat stress and enhance focus. Curiosity mingled with skepticism as she read stories of others who had experienced transformative effects. Could this be the answer she had been seeking?

As the days rolled on, Natalie decided to give Rhodiola a try. Each morning, she mixed the powder into her smoothie, savoring the earthy taste while hopeful thoughts danced through her mind. With every sip, she imagined herself gliding through her exams with confidence, her mind sharp and ready to tackle any question that came her way. But as exam day loomed closer, the familiar knot of anxiety tightened in her stomach.

The night before her first exam, sleep eluded her. Doubt whispered insidiously, questioning her decision to trust Rhodiola's promise of serenity. Would it really be enough? How could a mere herb soothe the storm brewing inside her? Each tick of the clock felt like a taunt, pulling her deeper into a whirlwind of worry. As she closed her eyes, the chaotic thoughts swirled, threatening to drown her amidst the tide of uncertainty.

The morning of the exam arrived, bringing with it a palpable tension. Despite her commitment to Rhodiola, irritation creased her brow as she surveyed her stacked textbooks. She felt unprepared, acutely aware of the glaring gap between her expectations and the reality of her knowledge. But as she clutched her pen, she noticed a hint of calmness begin to unfurl within her. Rhodiola had dulled the edge of her anxiety, allowing a flicker of hope to ignite.

But just as she began to breathe, her heart raced—she recalled the critical concepts she had glossed over in her studies. Panic surged, wrapping its icy fingers around her. Would Rhodiola's effects hold up when push came to shove? As she flipped the exam booklet, the questions stared back at her like predators waiting to pounce. Could she really advance into this test unscathed? She pressed her fingers against the cool surface of the desk, grounding herself as she fought against the impending storm within.

Natalie took a deep breath, letting the earthy aroma of Rhodiola linger in her mind as a potential anchor. But with each question, the tension mounted, her confidence wavering like a candle in the wind. Would this herbal ally be enough to guide her through the shadows of self-doubt? Heart pounding, she fought to focus—the stakes were high, and the outcome lay just out of reach.

Ashwagandha: Balancing Cortisol Levels

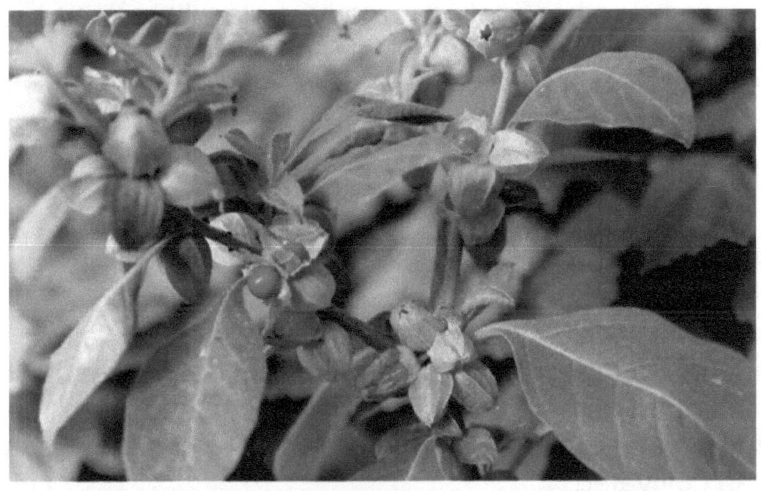

Oliver found himself staring blankly at his computer screen, the flickering cursor mirroring the chaos within his mind. The demands of his job often wrapped around him like a tight constriction, pressing against his chest with an unrelenting grip. He had heard whispers of a potent herb, Ashwagandha, said to combat stress and lower cortisol levels—the hormone that had become his uninvited companion. That evening, after yet another overwhelming day, he decided it was time to take control.

As Oliver researched, he uncovered stories of countless individuals who had experienced transformations thanks to Ashwagandha—a simple herb rooted deeply in the ancient practices of Ayurveda. With its ability to fixate on the very source of stress, it became clear that this herbal ally might be the answer he was seeking. He imagined awakening each morning feeling lighter, as if the weight of his work was merely a shadow fading in the light of dawn.

He hesitated for a moment, contemplating the upcoming stressors of next week's big presentation. What if Ashwagandha wouldn't work for him? What if it was just another fleeting remedy, a placebo promising relief but delivering none? Yet, an instinctive hope flickered within him, urging him to try. With a resolute heart, he ordered a supply of Ashwagandha capsules, refusing to surrender to the shadows of doubt.

Days passed and Oliver diligently integrated Ashwagandha into his routine. With each dose, he would find moments of calm amidst the spiraling confusion of deadlines and responsibilities. He felt a change, a new clarity filtering through the incessant noise. But as he prepared for his presentation, anxiety surged anew, threatening to drown out the tranquility he had cultivated.

On the day of the presentation, Oliver stood in front of his colleagues, palms clammy and heart racing. Doubt wrapped around him once again, but he sensed the whisper of Ashwagandha's promise lingering in the back of his mind. With every word he spoke, he envisioned shedding layers of stress, transforming into a more confident version of himself. But just as he reached the pivotal point of his pitch, his thoughts cascaded into a discordant clamor, eclipsing the hard-won peace he had forged.

What if the herb wasn't enough? What if, after all this, he still stumbled? As the minutes ticked by, the weight of expectation sharpened the air, and he realized that true balance went beyond the mere ingestion of a supplement. It demanded accountability to himself and the skills he had honed through relentless practice and dedication.

In that moment, Oliver grasped that perhaps Ashwagandha was not simply about alleviating stress; it was also about embarking on a deeper journey of self-belief and control. He took a deep breath, channeling the essence of all he had learned—about the herb, about the mind, and about navigating his own fears. With his voice steadier, he pressed on, determined not just to survive, but to thrive.

As the presentation concluded, applause filled the room, a sound drowned in a rush of relief and self-acceptance. Oliver had balanced his cortisol levels, not only with Ashwagandha but with the understanding that mastering his mind meant tackling the roots of his anxiety head-on. He had embraced the tension, confronting it with newfound strength, ready to face whatever came next.

Bacopa Monnieri: Memory Booster

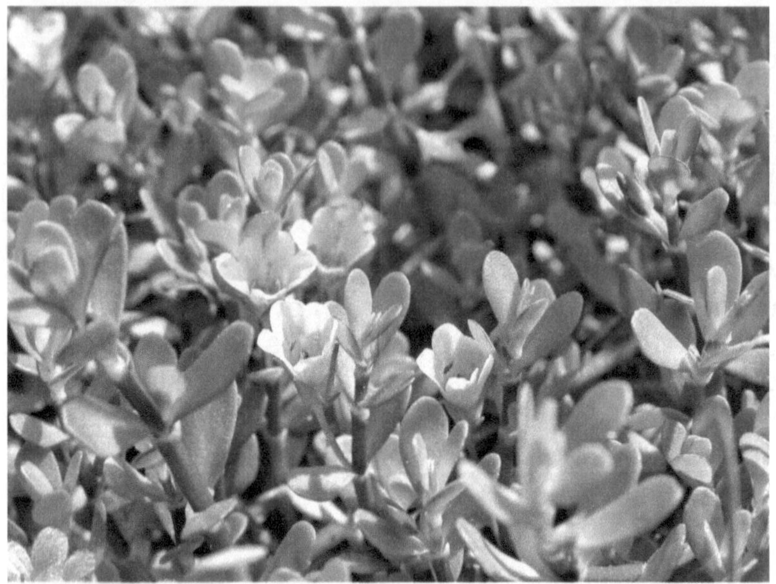

Sophie had always struggled with retaining information, especially during her hectic college years. As she rummaged through her backpack, searching for her notes before the big exam, a small bottle caught her eye—Bacopa Monnieri. She had read about its memory-enhancing properties online and decided to give it a try, hoping for the academic breakthrough she'd desperately needed.

With the morning sun streaming through her window, Sophie poured herself a glass of water and took the supplement, believing this might be the key to unlocking her potential. However, little did she know that this simple act would be the beginning of a profound journey. As days turned into weeks, Sophie began experiencing shifts that felt almost mystical, transforming her study sessions into an exhilarating chase of knowledge and retention.

Yet, as her memory improved, so did the pressure she felt from her peers and self-imposed expectations. The weight of ambition bore down on her, creating an internal tension that clashed with her newfound clarity. Late one evening, surrounded by textbooks and a mountain of flashcards, a nagging fear crept into her heart. What if this memory enhancement was merely a facade? What if it only served to amplify her struggle, rather than alleviate it?

With every bit of information she absorbed, shadows loomed larger over her confidence. Sophie began to question if she could maintain this momentum or if the inevitable crash was lurking around the corner. As exam day approached, her mind fluctuated between elation and dread, an emotional rollercoaster threatening to derail her progress.

Finally, the night before the exam arrived. With Bacopa on the table beside her, Sophie faced the momentary stillness punctuated by the ticking of the clock. All the knowledge she had gathered flitted in and out of her mind like a restless ghost. Would the supplement truly stand by her side when it mattered most? As she grappled with her thoughts, the tension was palpable, and the fear of failure clawed at her heart.

In that moment, Sophie made a choice. She closed her eyes and took a deep breath, letting the fears and doubts slip away like sand through her fingers. With the promise of Bacopa whispering a subtle assurance, she decided to trust in herself, ready to rise to the occasion, but aware now that the battle was not just about memory—it was a quest for inner peace amidst chaos.

The Impact of Lifestyle

Exercise: Moving for the Mind

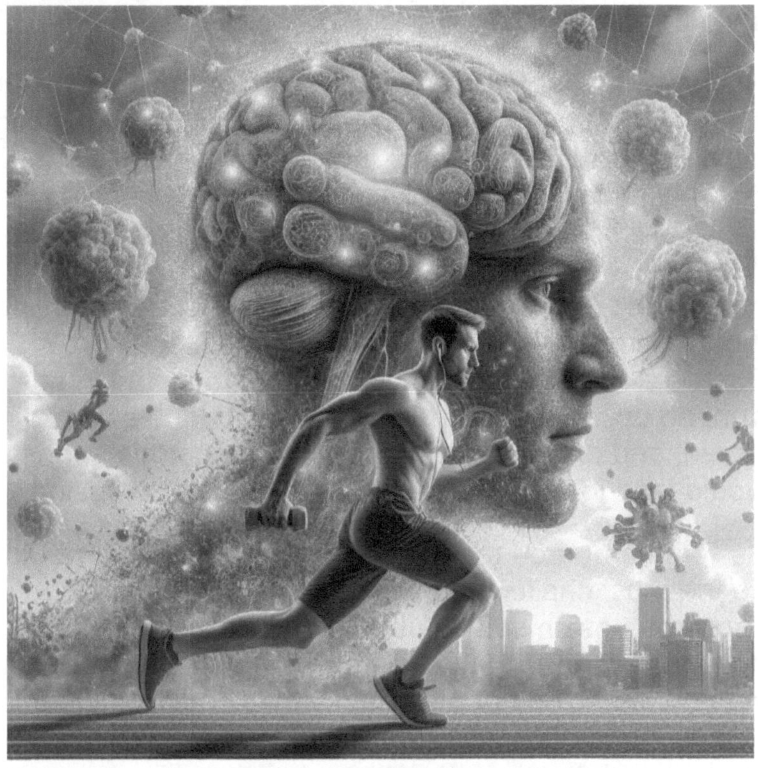

Ryan had always considered exercise a chore, something to fit in between the demands of his work and daily life. But as he embarked on this journey toward cognitive health, he began to realize there was more at stake than just physical fitness. The scientific studies that once seemed abstract took on new meaning; moving his body could mean better memory, sharper focus, and an enhanced overall sense of well-being.

With every morning jog and each visit to the gym, he felt a growing sense of clarity taking shape within him. The endorphins surged, flooding his brain with a wave of positivity that propelled him forward. He started to notice the little things—like how colors seemed more vibrant and conversations with colleagues flowed more easily. The fog that had lingered over his mind began to lift, not entirely, but enough for him to catch glimpses of a clearer horizon.

However, as he delved deeper, Ryan discovered that it wasn't just about moving his body; it was about moving his mind as well. It became imperative for him to seek out challenges that provoked thought while pushing his physical limits. The more he conditioned himself to face difficulties head-on in his workouts, the more resilient he became in everyday scenarios. But soon, a nagging thought crept in—was he pushing himself too hard? Each set and every mile was a test, and as the intensity ramped up, so did his anxiety. It was a double-edged sword, and only time would reveal whether his efforts would lead to enlightenment or just further confusion.

As Ryan prepared for what he promised himself would be the most challenging workout yet, an indomitable sense of tension settled upon him. The clock ticked ominously, shouting the hours away, and with each second, that cloud of uncertainty thickened. Would this dedication to his physicality yield the mental clarity he so desperately sought? With his heart racing and palms clammy, he took a deep breath—this was more than just exercise; it was a crossroads moment that could determine the trajectory of his cognitive health journey.

Sleep: The Forgotten Element

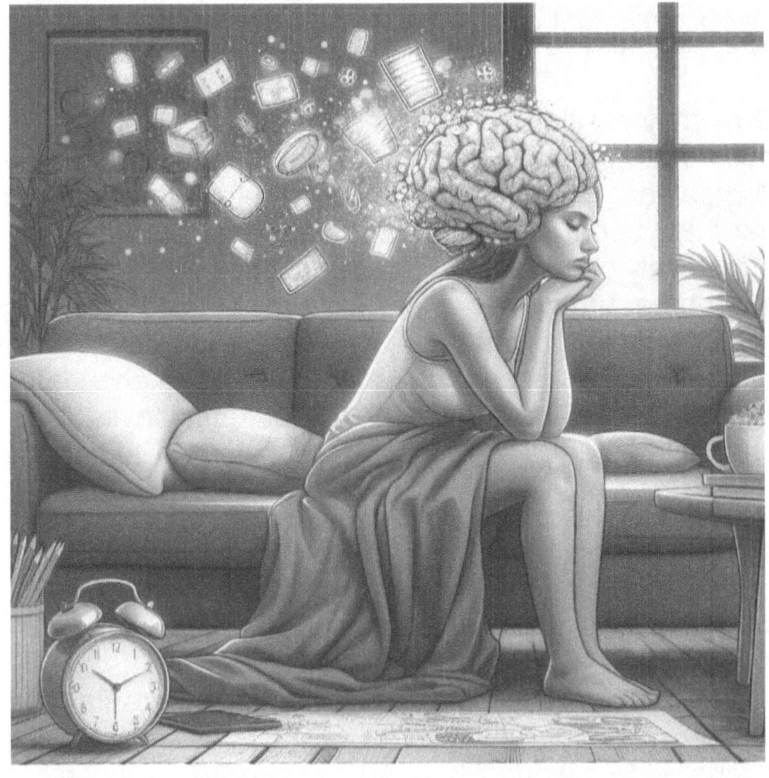

Claire paced back and forth in her small apartment, her mind racing with the myriad of tasks her life demanded. With deadlines looming and exams approaching, the idea of sacrificing sleep for productivity seemed almost inevitable. Yet, deep down, she felt a nagging suspicion that this strategy was flawed. As summer approached, the sun lingered longer in the sky, but Claire's nights grew darker, her body yearning for rest yet blinded by ambition.

During a particularly exhausting week, Claire stumbled upon a podcast that discussed the critical role of sleep in cognitive function. The host spoke with a blend of authority and understanding, weaving in stories of individuals who traded their dreams for screens, only to find themselves grappling with memory lapses and unexplainable fatigue. Intrigued yet apprehensive, Claire realized that perhaps she'd underestimated sleep, viewing it only as a luxury rather than the necessity it truly was.

Driven by her desire to succeed, Claire resolved to push through; sleep deprivation became her silent companion. However, as the days melded into weeks, her mind began to falter. Information that once flowed effortlessly became a patchwork of confusion. It felt as though her brain was a busy highway choked with traffic, unable to yield to clarity. Panic began to set in as her beloved study sessions turned into futile encounters with textbooks, words swirling like autumn leaves caught in a gust.

As she sought solace in caffeine and adrenaline, a shadow loomed over her efforts. It wasn't just her grades at stake; it was the very foundation of her cognitive health. Was it too late to prioritize rest? Doubt crept in, and with each passing sleepless night, the prospect of a restful sleep felt like a distant dream, tantalizing but perpetually out of reach. Claire felt anchored to a world where success relied solely on wakefulness—a haunting reflection of her priorities, threatening to consume her.

Then, one fateful evening, at the urging of a concerned friend, Claire decided to take a break. She shut her laptop, closed her books, and ventured into the fresh air—the kind of air that filled her lungs with possibility. That walk turned into an epiphany as she began to consider the profound impact sleep had on her memory and focus. The thought bloomed into determination: could she reclaim her nights? What if she wove rest into her routine as earnestly as she pursued her studies?

Excitement stirred within her; however, fear began to mingle with that excitement. Could she really abstain from studying late? Would the pressure of her academic career allow her to prioritize sleep? As her plan materialized, a wave of uncertainty crashed over her, accompanied by an equally potent resolve. Claire knew this was not merely about adding sleep; it was about transforming her approach to success. She began to chart her path—a delicate balance she hoped would foster respect for her body's needs while still demanding brilliance from her mind.

Yet, as the impending deadline loomed, Claire felt the tug of anxiety pull her back to old habits. Torn between the whisper of restful sleep and the siren call of her ambition, she stood at a precipice, poised to leap into a new way of living. There was a promise of clarity on the horizon, but the question remained: would she allow herself to embrace it, or would she slip back into the chaotic abyss of sleepless nights, forever haunted by the shadows of her unfulfilled potential?

Mindfulness: The Power of Presence

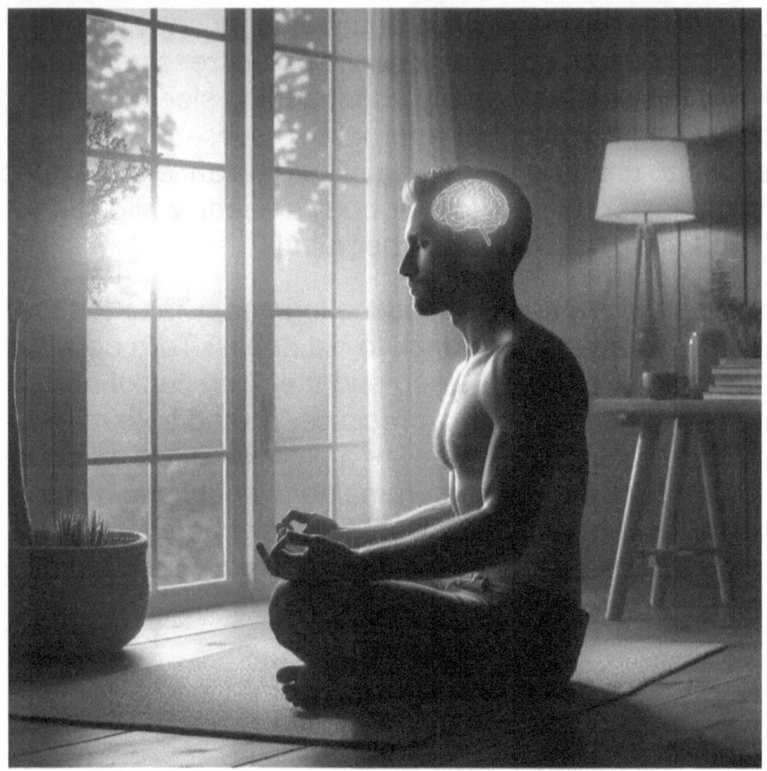

As David embarked on his mindfulness journey, he found himself seated in his quiet corner of the world, a gentle hum of morning outside his window. The soft light illuminated the room, creating a safe space where he could explore the depths of his thoughts. Invoking the principles of mindfulness, he began to focus on his breathing, each inhale a step towards clarity, each exhale a release of tension that seemed to cloud his mind.

But the real challenge lay beyond the serene folds of his surroundings. David couldn't escape the mounting pressures of his daily life—the endless deadlines, the swirling chaos of his thoughts, and the self-imposed expectations that often left him overwhelmed. He learned quickly that mindfulness wasn't merely about quiet moments of reflection; it involved confronting the very stressors that pushed him beyond the limits of his mental capacity.

Delving deeper into mindfulness, David incorporated simple techniques into his routine: he began to practice body scans, noticing how tension accumulated in unexpected parts—his shoulders and jaw, remnants of an unseen weight he carried. He embraced guided meditations, each session a compass guiding him back to the present. Yet, as days turned into weeks, unsettling feelings crept in. The very act of being present forced him to confront emotions he had long suppressed. Gradually, the power of presence revealed both the beauty and the discomfort of his inner landscape.

One gloomy afternoon, sitting cross-legged with eyes closed, David felt an unusual heaviness swallow him whole. Images of past failures and anxieties flooded his mind, pulling him into a spiral of self-doubt. It was at that moment he realized that mindfulness was not a panacea; it was a mirror reflecting back the struggles he fought to hide. The tension escalated within him as he grappled with this revelation, leaving him teetering on the verge of panic.

Beneath the unwavering facade of composure he had cultivated, a tempest of emotions raged. Could he truly embrace the present when the present felt so heavy? With each breath, uncertainty hovered like an ominous cloud, threatening to unleash a storm. In that critical moment, David had a choice: to retreat back into old patterns or to lean into the discomfort, trusting that perhaps the greatest power of presence lay not in avoidance, but in unconditional acceptance of his current experience.

Navigating the Market

Choosing Quality Supplements

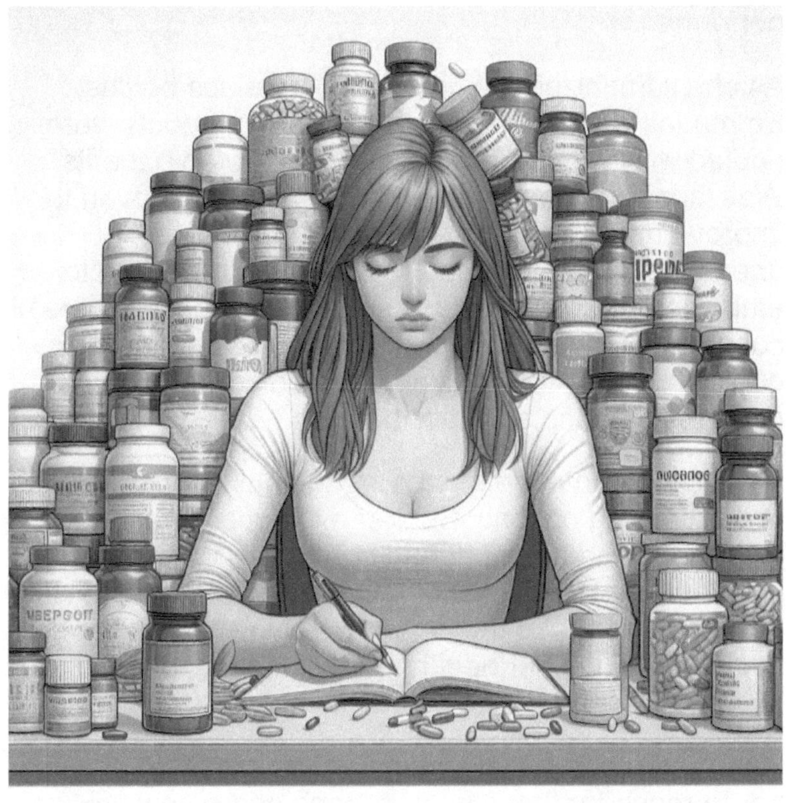

Emma sat at her desk, surrounded by a seemingly endless array of supplement bottles, each promising to enhance her cognitive prowess. As a student, the pressure to excel was ever-present, and she was determined to find the right combination of supplements that would give her the edge she needed. But with so many options flooding the market, how could she be certain she was making the right choice?

She began her research by prioritizing quality over quantity. Chatting with friends and seeking advice from online forums led her to recognize the importance of reputable brands. "If a supplement is too cheap to be true, it probably is," she recalled her friend's sage advice. With this mantra in mind, Emma delved deeper into the labyrinth of labels, deciphering which ingredients truly mattered for maximizing her mental performance.

As she scrutinized the fine print on various bottles, Emma felt a pang of frustration. Many products were riddled with vague claims and exaggerated benefits. Was 'supports brain function' the same as 'proven to improve memory'? The ambiguity left her feeling uneasy, but she pressed on, fueled by the desire to empower herself with knowledge. After hours of careful comparison, she developed a checklist to identify quality supplements: full ingredient disclosure, third-party testing, and scientific backing.

Working late into the night, Emma finally honed in on a few promising options. But her excitement was soon overshadowed by doubt and confusion. What if her choices didn't work? What if they had adverse effects? She couldn't shake the inner voice whispering that she might be risking her health in pursuit of academic success.

Her heart raced as she imagined the pressure causing her to reach for those bottles, each one a new risk waiting to unfold. Suddenly, she realized that her journey was about more than just enhancing her cognitive abilities; it was about making informed decisions aligned with her wellness goals. Emma took a deep breath, determined to stick to her checklist and choose supplements wisely. As she prepared to place her first order, the weight of her choices loomed large, and uncertainty lingered heavily in the air.

Understanding Labels and Claims

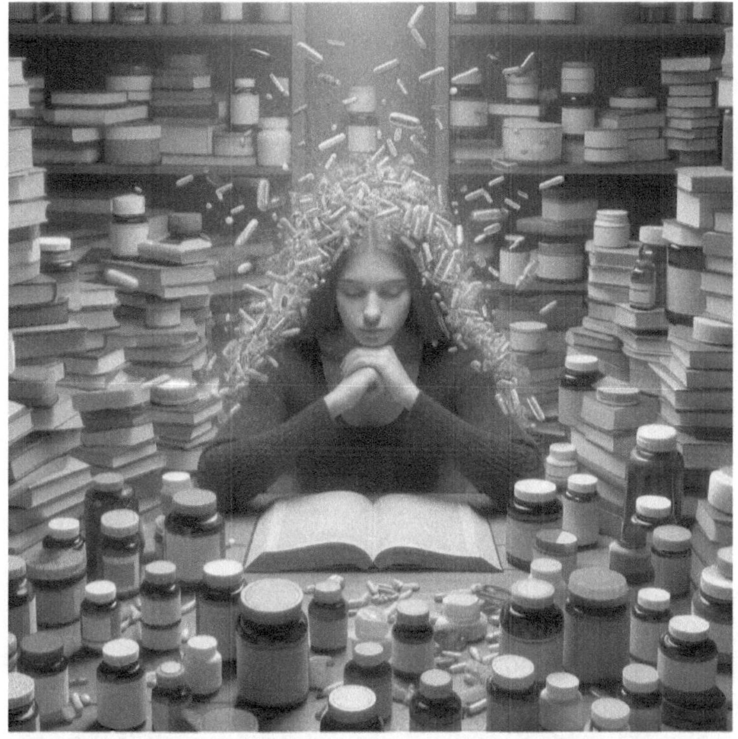

In a marketplace flooded with choices, Emma felt the weight of her decision-making burdening her like a heavy backpack. Each bottle and box screamed for her attention with bright labels and bold claims. She reminded herself that understanding these labels was essential, for her cognitive health depended on the choices she made.

As she dove deeper into the world of supplements, she learned that not all products were created equal. Powered by curiosity, she began to decode the jargon that danced across the packaging. 'No artificial ingredients,' ' clinically tested,' and 'proven efficacy'—each phrase seemed to promise a gateway to enhanced cognitive performance. Yet, beneath the surface, a labyrinth of misinformation loomed. Emma's heart raced as she questioned the validity of each claim, fearful of falling victim to clever marketing tactics.

Her late-night research sessions ensued, where she poured over scientific articles and expert reviews, seeking clues that could guide her through the confusion. She started to understand that supplements were not a magic bullet; they were just one piece of a much larger puzzle. A sense of urgency grew within her, a longing not just for knowledge but for empowerment. Could she truly trust the face value of these products? As doubts crept in, Emma knew she had to stand firm in her pursuit of truth, determined to navigate this complex landscape without losing her way.

Then, just as she was piecing together her newfound wisdom, a friend shared a concerning article about counterfeit supplements infiltrating reputable brands. Emma's pulse quickened—how could she ever be sure of what she was consuming? The pressure mounted as she felt the enormity of her responsibility not only to herself but also to her fragile aspirations. She was on the verge of something exhilarating, yet perilously close to a misstep that could derail her journey entirely.

Armed with a list of trusted resources, Emma braced herself to face the aisles of product confusion again. The tension hung thick in the air as she approached the shelves, her heart pounding with each step. In that moment, she realized that navigating the market was not just about choosing products; it was also about understanding herself, reclaiming her power, and standing resilient in a world that often thrives on uncertainty.

The Importance of Research

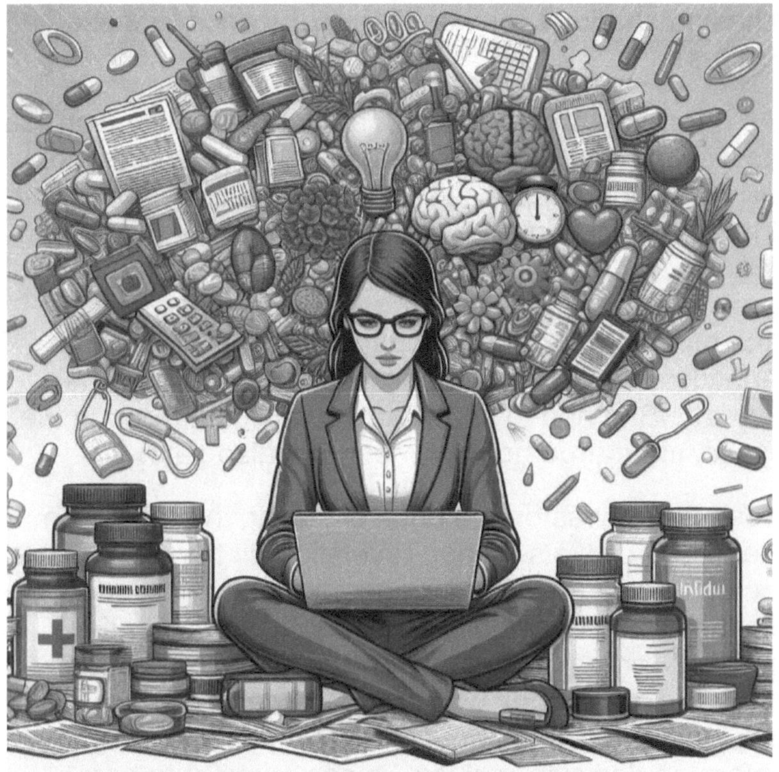

Samantha found herself in a world teeming with information, symbols, and promises—each supplement vying for her attention, each label shouting its own truth. It was here, in this cacophony, that she realized the necessity of stepping back and discerning the facts from the fables. Armed with a laptop and a determination fueled by her growing curiosity, she began her expedition into the realm of cognitive health supplements.

But as she delved deeper, the tension within her began to rise. Certain articles contradicted others, clouding her quest for clarity. Just when she thought she understood the complex web of neurotransmitters and their relationship to cognitive function, she stumbled upon testimonials laden with promises but devoid of scientific backing. Gradually, doubt crept in; was she chasing shadows, or was there substance to these claims?

As her research progressed, a nagging feeling wormed its way into her thoughts—what if she were to gamble on the wrong supplement, one that could wreak havoc instead of helping her? A sense of urgency mingled with her determination. It pushed her to reach out to professionals in the field, to engage in forums, where like-minded seekers shared their stories. Yet, scary anecdotes mingled with success stories, fueling her anxiety. She had to find a way to navigate through the noise, to emerge not just wiser, but also safe.

Just as she was on the brink of pulling the trigger on her first order, a sobering revelation hit her: she might be entangled in a world far deeper than anticipated, a field evolving constantly and fraught with potential pitfalls. Samantha closed her laptop, taking a deep breath. This journey was not merely about choosing a supplement; it was about embracing a lifestyle of informed decision-making—a commitment to her cognitive future. The stakes were high, and she needed to tread carefully.

Little did she know that the ultimate test of her research was just around the corner, waiting for her to uncover. As she gathered the courage to move forward, the shadows of doubt whispering in her ear grew louder, warning her of the challenges lurking just beyond the path she was ready to tread.

Personal Stories

The Student's Perspective

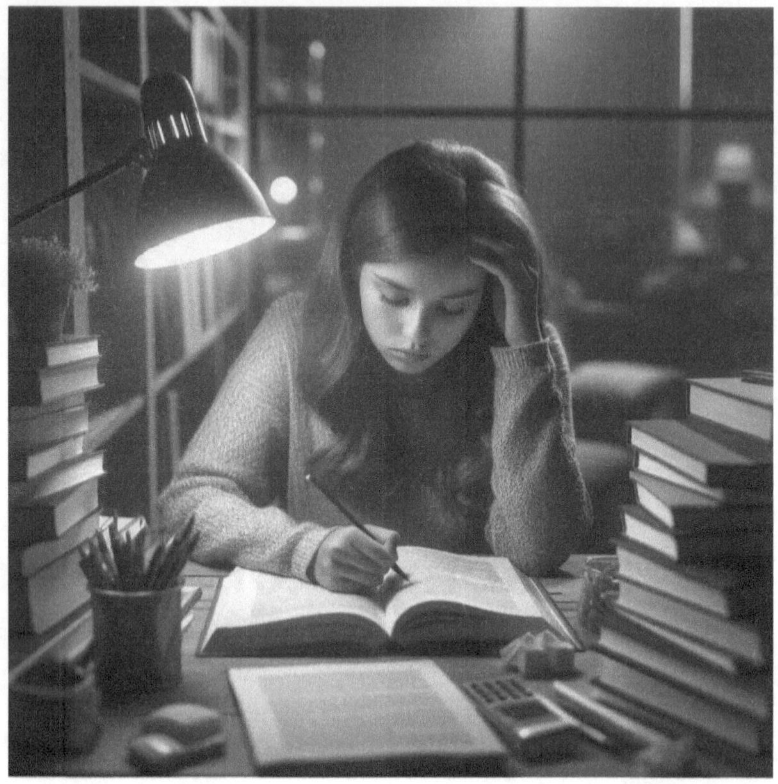

Heather sat at her desk, the soft glow of the desk lamp illuminating her textbooks scattered around her. With finals week approaching, she felt the familiar pressure mounting, a whirlwind of anxiety mixed with determination. It was a typical evening, but there was more at stake. This time, she had decided to take a different approach toward her study routine—an approach that involved cognitive support through dietary changes and supplements.

After hearing about the cognitive benefits of Omega-3 fatty acids and B vitamins, Heather dove headfirst into research. She explored various blog posts and scientific articles, learning how these nutrients could enhance memory and focus. However, the more she learned the more disheartening it became; each piece of information revealed not just potential benefits but the likelihood of failure if she didn't integrate them into her routine consistently. The weight of expectation pressed down on her shoulders, and she found herself questioning if the investment in these supplements would truly make a difference in her stressed-out student life.

As days turned into nights filled with cramming, Heather could feel the urgency turning into desperation. On one particularly frustrating evening, she glanced at the bottle of Ginkgo Biloba she had purchased but rarely used. If I just stick to it, she murmured to herself, maybe it will sharpen my focus. With that thought lingering in her mind, she took a deep breath and made a commitment: to approach her studies with purpose armed with the power of nutrients and a newfound belief in her ability to succeed.

As Heather's exam dates loomed ever closer, she implemented her plan, incorporating the supplements into her daily routine. It felt empowering at first, but as the reality of her dwindling time sank in, self-doubt crept in, whispering that it might all be for naught. The tension grew as classmates began sharing their strategies and study materials in the chat group, each message a reminder of her own insecurities about the choices she had made. The looming specter of failure hung over her, threatening to disrupt the careful balance she had built. Would the supplements be enough? Or would they only become another added layer of stress in her already chaotic life?

With just days left until the exams, Heather's resolve began to waver. During a late-night study session, the pressure reached a boiling point as she struggled to retain crucial details. She stood up abruptly, her chair scraping across the wooden floor, and paced around her room, overwhelmed. Frustration bubbled over as she started to doubt everything—the supplements, the late nights, even her own capabilities.

In that moment of despair, she received a message from a fellow student, sharing their own struggles and the feeling of hopelessness they experienced while studying. It struck a chord within Heather; suddenly, she was reminded that she was not alone in this journey. Perhaps the camaraderie of shared experiences might just be the catalyst she needed to harness her resolve once more. With renewed determination, she took a deep breath, sat back down, and prepared to tackle one last round of studying, her heart pounding with a mix of fear and hope.

A Professional's Journey

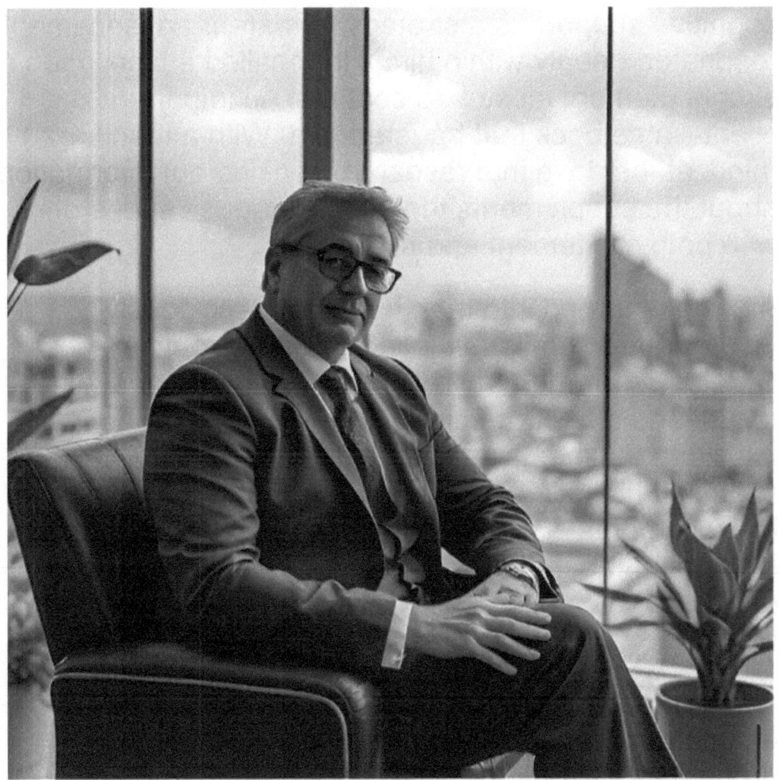

Tom sat in his corner office, the city skyline visible through the expansive glass windows. The world seemed to move at a frantic pace outside, but inside, he felt ensnared in his own thoughts, struggling to keep up with the demands of a fast-paced corporate environment. Despite his accomplishments, the weight of expectations bore down on him, and he knew something had to change. His journey toward cognitive support began inexplicably during a particularly stressful quarter when performance metrics were at an all-time low.

Initially skeptical about the role of nutritional supplements in enhancing cognitive capabilities, Tom gradually opened himself to the idea after attending a seminar where industry leaders shared their own stories of transformation. The concept of utilizing cognitive support as a strategy for career advancement resonated deeply within him. He recalled a time when a simple memory lapse had cost him an important client—a setback that haunted him. With a resolute mindset, he dove into research, seeking out information about the supplements that his colleagues spoke of with both excitement and reverence.

As weeks turned into months, Tom meticulously incorporated supplements into his daily routine—Omega-3s for memory retention, Ginkgo Biloba for focus, and a multivitamin to fill in the gaps. Every day felt like a battle against distractions that had once shackled him. He began to notice subtle improvements—conversations flowed more naturally, ideas sparked more readily, and he found himself re-engaging with colleagues in ways he had long thought lost.

However, as he climbed higher in his career, he encountered unexpected obstacles. New projects brought increased responsibility and a heightened sense of pressure. Just as Tom started feeling in control of his cognitive health, he faced a nerve-wracking challenge: a pivotal presentation looming on the horizon. The stakes were higher than ever, and the shadow of self-doubt crept in, whispering that perhaps he hadn't changed at all, that he was merely living a charade. He grappled with the fear of slipping back into oblivion, questioning whether cognitive support could truly save him from the impending storm.

On the night before the presentation, Tom paced, his thoughts spiraling. His carefully curated strategies felt awash in uncertainty. In the dim light of his office, he reached for his journal—a compilation of notes detailing his journey. Each page echoed raw moments of vulnerability, resilience, and the unwavering desire for success. As he read, a spark ignited within him, fanning the flames of his determination. He had come too far to let fear rob him of the progress he had worked so diligently to achieve.

With resolve filling him anew, Tom embraced the significance of both his cognitive health journey and the lessons learned from setbacks. The next day, he stood before his team, heart pounding yet firmly grounded by the knowledge and insights he had gleaned along the way. He welcomed the challenge, understanding now that it was not merely about the supplements or techniques, but about the unwavering courage to confront his fears head-on.

As he delivered his presentation, a blend of confidence and anxiety lifted him, the earlier doubts dissipating as the room filled with nodding heads and engaged faces. In that moment, Tom realized that the journey was far from over; it was merely the beginning of a lifelong commitment to nurturing his cognitive health amidst the triumphs and trials of professional life.

The Everyday Hero

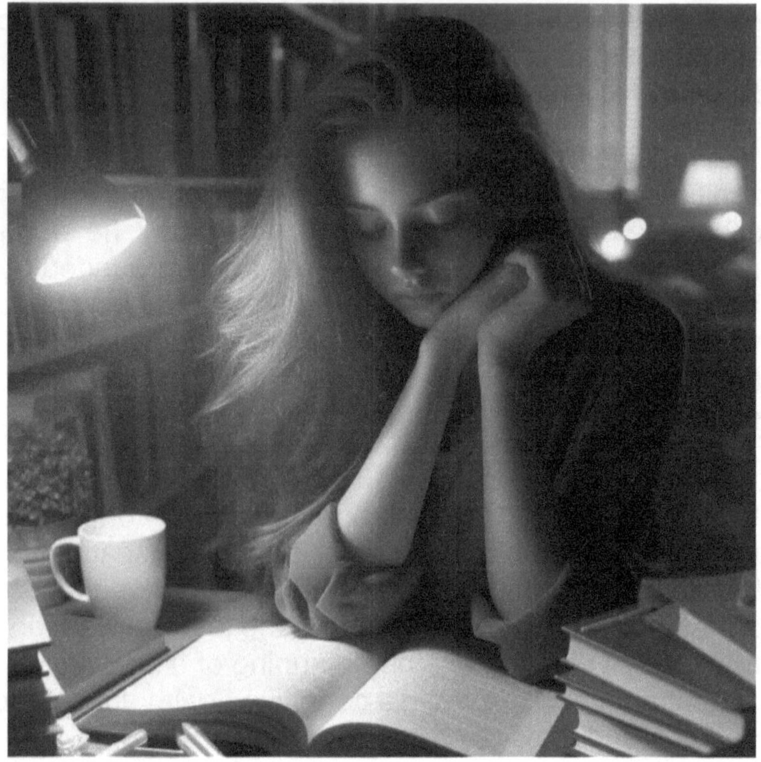

Maria always considered herself an ordinary person, juggling the demands of work, family, and her own aspirations. Amid the chaos of everyday life, she had begun to notice the toll it all took on her cognitive health. Mornings were bleary-eyed as she shuffled through her routine, often forgetting where she had placed her keys or losing track of conversations. It was a gradual decline, but she could feel it weighing heavily on her mind.

On one particularly overwhelming day, Maria had to help her son with his school project, prepare dinner for her family, and finish a report for work—all while also trying to squeeze in a quick workout. The stress was palpable, and her mind felt foggy. It was then that Maria realized she couldn't afford to let her cognitive health slip any further. Just as heroes had their calling, she felt it was time for her own personal transformation.

Determined to prioritize her cognitive wellbeing, Maria began researching supplements that could enhance her mental clarity and focus. She surrounded herself with resources, listened to experts, and joined online forums filled with others like her, eager for change. As she navigated this new path, each small step felt monumental—she started incorporating mindfulness practices and routine exercises into her life.

Yet, even as she made positive strides, there were days when doubt crept in during the quiet moments, gnawing at her resolve. Would it really make a difference? Was she strong enough to sustain these commitments? Then, just when the tension peaked, a sudden challenge emerged—a massive work project landed unexpectedly on her desk, demanding her full attention and significantly pressing her cognitive limits.

As deadlines loomed, the chaos surrounding Maria intensified. She was faced with a choice: revert back to her old habits, or lean into the cognitive practices she had been cultivating. Driven by the love for her family and the desire to be the best version of herself, Maria chose to honor her journey. It was a race against time, and she was determined to emerge stronger, wielding the tools she had gathered in the face of adversity.

With every ounce of strength, Maria pushed through the project, focusing on her training, her supplements, and her newfound mindfulness. As the deadline approached, the pressure mounted like never before. But amidst the chaos, she felt a flicker of hope—she realized she wasn't just a participant in her life; she was a hero, fighting to rewrite her story. Would her day of reckoning prove to be a triumphant victory or an insurmountable setback? The answer awaited on the other side of the impending deadline.

Building a Routine

Integrating Supplements into Daily Life

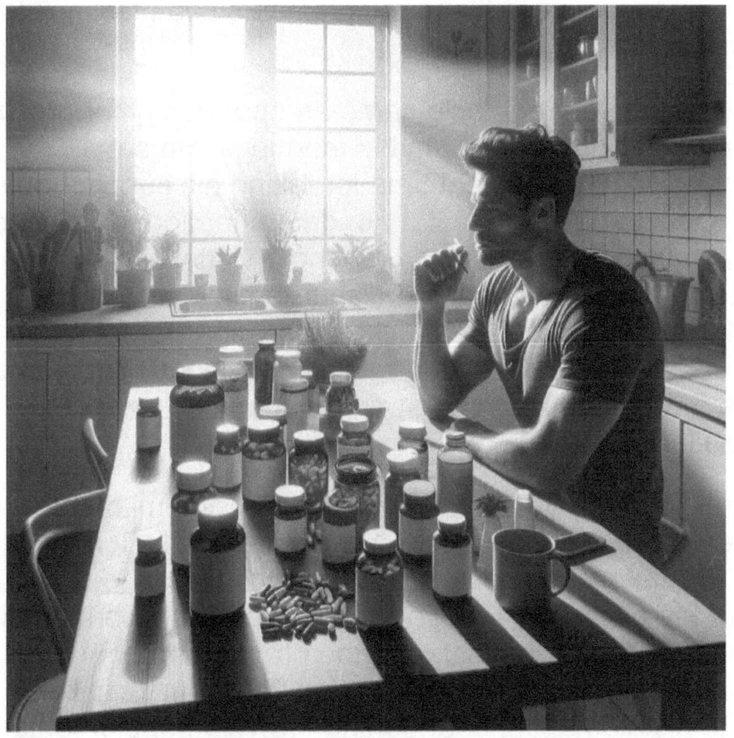

Kevin sat at his kitchen table, the morning sun streaming in, illuminating the array of bottles before him. Each capsule and powder promised something different, a solution to clarity, focus, and an energy boost to counter the morning drowsiness. It was a new commitment, a promise to himself to enhance his daily routine. But as he struggled to form a habit with his new supplements, doubts crept in: Would these really help him? Or were they just another distraction?

The transition from sporadic use to a solid routine was proving to be more challenging than he had anticipated. Each morning, he battled with the familiar voices in his head whispering doubts and distractions. After a few weeks, his enthusiasm began to wane. He found himself reaching for coffee more often, the supplements gathering dust, and his morning ritual felt less like a commitment and more like a chore. Would he ever find a way to integrate these supplements seamlessly into his life?

But with every obstacle came an opportunity for growth. Kevin decided to reclaim his mornings. He set a schedule: a consistent time for taking his supplements alongside his breakfast. With determination, he placed the bottles in plain sight, creating a visual reminder of his commitment. As the days turned into weeks, he started feeling the subtle changes—sharper focus at work, a clearer mind during study sessions. Yet, just as he thought he was on the right path, an unexpected challenge arose.

Amidst rising deadlines and personal commitments, Kevin experienced the all-too-familiar sensation of overwhelm. The noise of his daily life began to drown out the clarity he'd fought to achieve. Each work email piled on top of the last, and the pressures from both his job and social life felt suffocating. Would he slip back into his old habits, abandoning the very supplements that were meant to elevate him?

Harnessing his determination, he began to journal; a simple yet powerful way to track not just his supplement intake but also his thoughts and feelings. It helped keep him grounded, a lifeline amidst the chaos. Slowly, he learned not just to integrate the supplements effectively but to balance them against the myriad of stresses life threw his way. Then came that fateful day when Kevin woke up to an unexpected deadline looming over him—an important presentation he hadn't prepared for amidst his newfound routine.

With anxiety creeping in and doubts threatening to overwhelm him, he stood at a crossroads: would he allow the pressure to derail his progress or use it to rise above? As the clock ticked down towards his presentation, Kevin's heart raced, unsure if he could balance his new healthy habits with the mounting chaos of his responsibilities. Would he rise to the challenge or fall back into the shadows of a life not fully lived? The answer, he knew, lay just within reach if he dared to grasp it.

Setting Realistic Goals

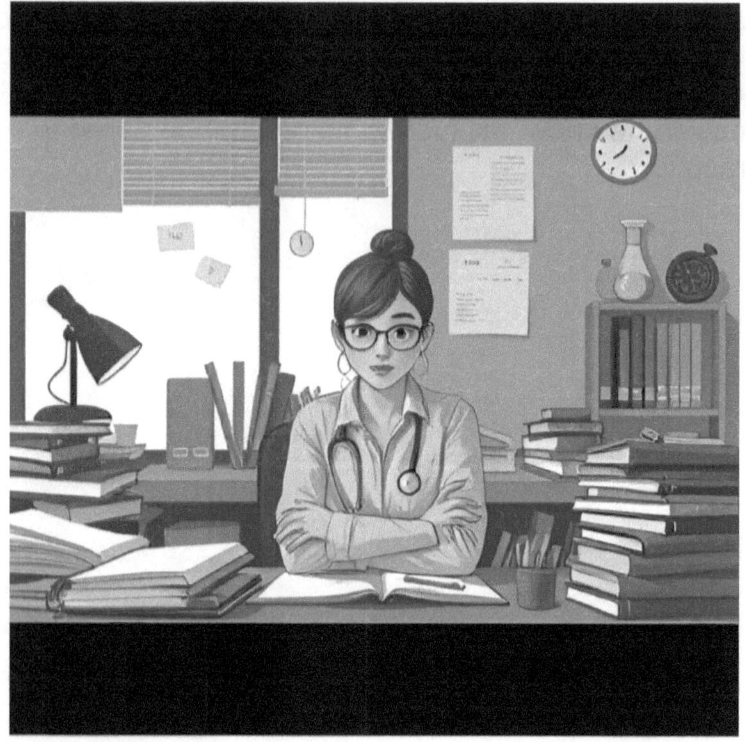

Sophie sat at her cluttered desk, surrounded by textbooks and notes, a mix of anxiety and determination swirling within her. She had recently realized that her cognitive abilities were not as sharp as she wanted them to be, and she felt an undeniable urge to change that. The pressure of looming exams and her desire to excel academically weighed heavily on her, reminding her that improvement wouldn't happen overnight. Setting realistic, achievable goals felt critical, yet daunting.

She began by breaking down her aspirations into smaller, manageable steps. Instead of simply declaring, I will improve my memory, she crafted a plan that included reading a chapter a day, practicing mnemonic devices, and dedicating time each week for review.

Each tiny aim felt like a small victory, and with a notepad in hand, she jotted them down. Yet, as the familiar wave of self-doubt washed over her, she wondered if these goals were ambitious enough or if they still fell short of her potential. The internal battle intensified.

With each goal she set, Sophie reminded herself to be gentle. While striving for greatness, she understood the importance of celebrating even the most minor milestones. Each memory technique mastered, each study session completed, and every ounce of progress deserved recognition. She envisioned herself months from now, perhaps sitting in a cozy café, confidently reviewing notes and prepared for exams. But as she glanced at her reflective notes, she couldn't shake the feeling that time was slipping away. Would her goals, no matter how realistic, truly transform her cognitive abilities? The tension mounted as the deadline approached, casting a shadow over her quiet resolve.

Tracking Progress and Adjustments

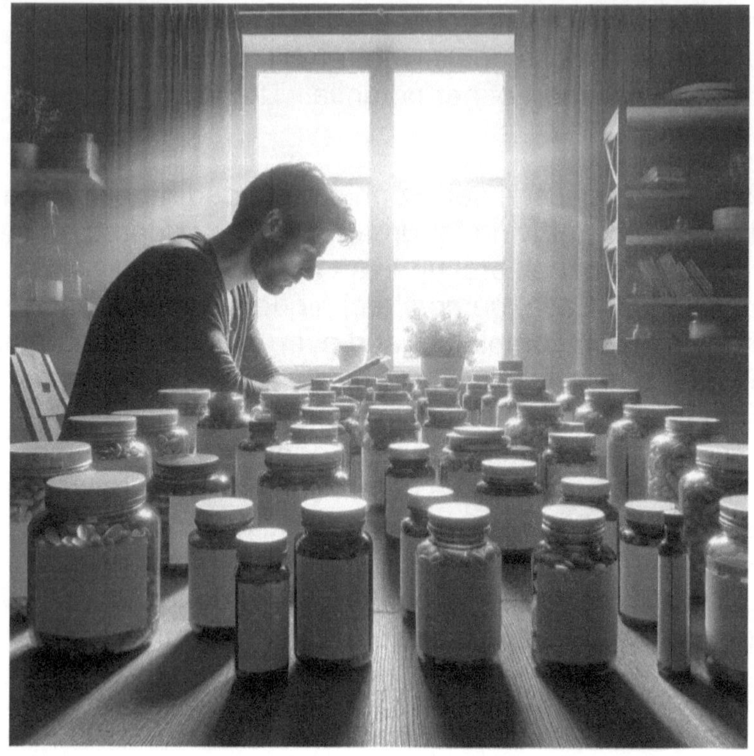

As Daniel embarked on his journey towards improved cognitive health, he quickly realized that simply following a regimen of supplements and lifestyle changes wasn't enough. He needed a way to track his progress, to see if his efforts were yielding tangible results. Each morning, as he sipped his green smoothie, he would jot down his thoughts in a journal—his accountability partner through the highs and lows of this quest.

Over time, Daniel established specific metrics to monitor his cognitive health: focus, energy levels, and even his memory recall. He developed a simple rating system, where 1 was "poor" and 5 was "excellent." But soon, self-reported measures began to feel insufficient. The inconsistency in his daily entries made him doubt his attempts at self-improvement; perhaps he wasn't changing at all. This frustration crept in like a dark cloud, casting doubt on his once-clear aspirations.

Determined to cut through the haze, Daniel sought other ways to measure his progress. He downloaded apps that provided cognitive tests, which offered a more objective glimpse into his mental performance. He meticulously logged his scores, taking note of fluctuations that mirrored the days he felt particularly engaged or, conversely, mentally drained. With each test, he felt the tension rise—what if he discovered he wasn't significantly improving? What if all his efforts were in vain?

One day, after a series of lackluster scores, an unexpected wave of anxiety washed over him. Daniel questioned the efficacy of the supplements and lifestyle changes he had so diligently incorporated, wondering if he should risk switching strategies entirely. Yet he knew that change wasn't always synonymous with progress. Could he truly be evolving if he wasn't yet seeing the results he envisioned?

As the weeks progressed, he found that his emotional responses to the tests varied greatly, depending on his mindset and the support he received from peers who were also on their cognitive journeys. He realized his own expectations and patience would need adjustments as well. Perhaps it was time to reflect, to engage in a deeper dialogue with himself about his aspirations.

And just as the weight of uncertainty threatened to overwhelm him, an unexpected realization broke through the fog: improvement is often a winding path, fraught with twists and turns, not a straight line. Armed with this new perspective, Daniel decided to embrace the journey more fully, allowing himself to celebrate small victories, even amidst setbacks. The inevitable highs and lows of progress became not just hurdles, but learning opportunities, reinvigorating his original motivation.

As he neared a pivotal moment in his journey, a sense of anticipation filled the air—would this renewed perspective lead to the breakthrough he sought? Or would it unravel the very progress he had begun to reclaim? The uncertainty lingered, charging the atmosphere with a palpable tension that left Daniel both hopeful and anxious, standing on the brink of transformation.

Cognitive Challenges

Identifying Cognitive Decline

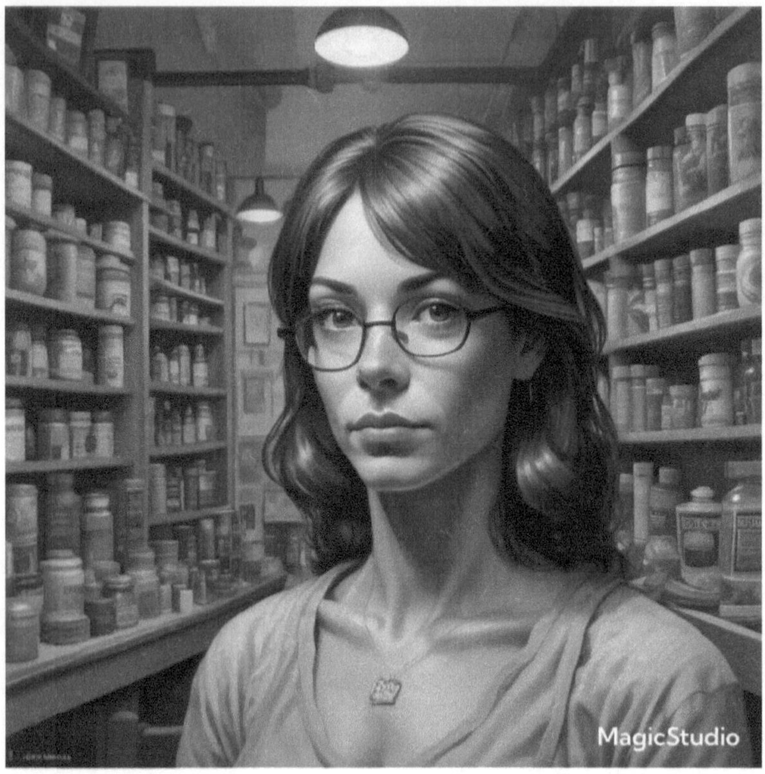

As Sarah settled into her new routine, she began to notice peculiar changes in her cognition that stirred a palpable fear within her. Tasks she once tackled with ease now felt overwhelmingly difficult, like navigating a dense fog without a guiding light. She often found herself forgetting simple things—where she placed her keys, the names of acquaintances she used to greet without hesitation. Each lapse in memory chipped away at her confidence, leaving her pondering the unsettling possibility of cognitive decline.

This realization prompted Sarah to embark on a quest for answers, a desperate need to understand what was happening to her mind. Armed with determination, she delved into research, seeking insights from renowned neurologists, reading countless articles, and even participating in online forums. Her heart raced with every article she consumed that hinted at early-stage cognitive decline, but she clung to hope the knowledge would lead her to a path of healing rather than despair.

Through her research, Sarah discovered various assessment tools designed to identify cognitive decline early, like cognition quizzes and memory challenges. But as she grappled with self-assessments, a nagging doubt crept in—what if the results were worse than she imagined? With each passing day, the weight of knowledge started to feel like a double-edged sword, arming her with insight yet rendering her vulnerable to the fear that clung like a shadow. The tension between hope and dread tightened around her as she contemplated her next steps.

In her darkest moments, Sarah reached out to others, sharing her thoughts with friends and family, who offered a mixture of reassurance and concern. Their eyes reflected the empathy she desperately needed, yet she sensed their uncertainty. As she listened to their well-meaning advice—slow down, take it easy— she felt the pressure of unspoken expectations weigh heavily on her shoulders. Would they still see the capable, engaged person they had always known, or was she already becoming a shadow of her former self?

The urge to seek professional help grew stronger as her fear mounted. She scheduled a visit with a neurologist, apprehension coiling in her stomach as the appointment drew closer. What if she learned the truth she wasn't ready to face? What if this was just the beginning of a long, uncertain journey? The clock ticked steadily toward the date, each second amplifying her unease while igniting an unwavering resolve to not just accept what was happening, but to confront it head-on with every tool at her disposal.

As the day approached, the distinction between fear and proactivity blurred, pushing her to explore options beyond medical assessments—lifestyle changes, diet improvements, supplements that promised to reinforce her cognitive barriers. A rush of information flooded her mind as she juggled solutions and strategy, yet a part of her hesitated, fearing it might be too late to turn back the tide of decline. With courage gathering like a storm within her, Sarah braced herself for the appointment, knowing she was at a precipice where clarity awaited—along with the potential reality she had feared to confront.

The Role of Supplements in Aging

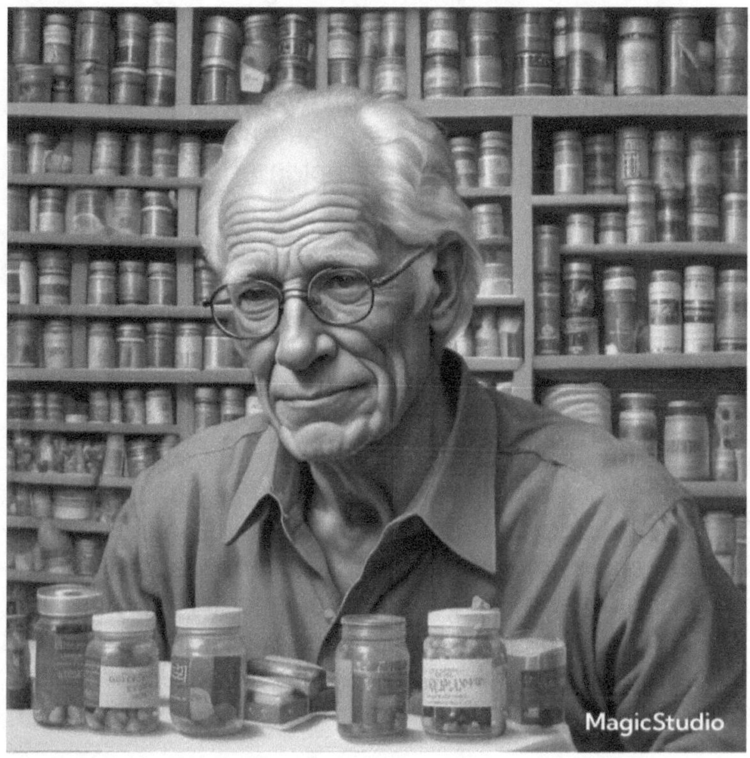

George had always prided himself on his sharp mind. The days of youthful vigor, filled with quick thinking and a memory that retained facts with ease, were once the foundation of his identity. But as the years progressed, he began to notice subtle changes—forgotten names, misplaced keys, and an occasional struggle to articulate thoughts. The creeping nature of aging sparked an urgent need for solutions, especially as his friends started voicing similar concerns about their cognitive health.

One evening, while sipping herbal tea, George discovered a promising article about supplements designed to support cognitive function in older adults. It piqued his interest, suggesting that certain nutrients could safeguard against the mental decline that often accompanied aging. Flashes of hope ignited within him as he researched names like Omega-3 fatty acids and B vitamins, learning how they purportedly worked miracles for the brain, enhancing memory and focus. Each article he read was filled with testimonials—individuals who had reclaimed their mental clarity simply by integrating these supplements into their daily routines.

Determined to take action, George devised a plan. With newfound vigor, he went on a quest to source high-quality supplements. His weekly trips to the local health store became a ritual, each visit an exhilarating exploration of new options. He started reminding himself that age was just a number, and every supplement was a small step toward regaining control. Yet, as he began incorporating them into his life, he couldn't shake the nagging fear that perhaps he was just grasping at straws in an ever-accelerating decline. Little did he know that the journey had just begun, and the path ahead would be filled with unexpected trials and revelations that were anything but easy.

One day, after several weeks of supplement intake, George was alarmed to face a particularly vivid episode of confusion. He was hosting friends for dinner when, in the middle of a story, his mind went blank. Anxiety washed over him as laughter echoed around the table—everyone else lost in joy while he was entrapped in a fog. Doubt crept in, and with it, the harsh realization that cognitive decline was more than just an idea; it was becoming his reality. The sharpness he once knew was faltering, replaced by an unsettling cloud of uncertainty.

As he sat in silence, listening to his friends' laughter, George felt an urge to delve deeper into his supplementation journey. It wasn't enough to simply consume; he needed to understand the science behind these choices. What guarantees did he have that they were effective against the unavoidable decline? At that moment, George vowed to not only remain steadfast in his supplement routine but to seek knowledge and community support, hoping to navigate the murky waters of cognitive change.

Addressing ADHD and Focus Issues

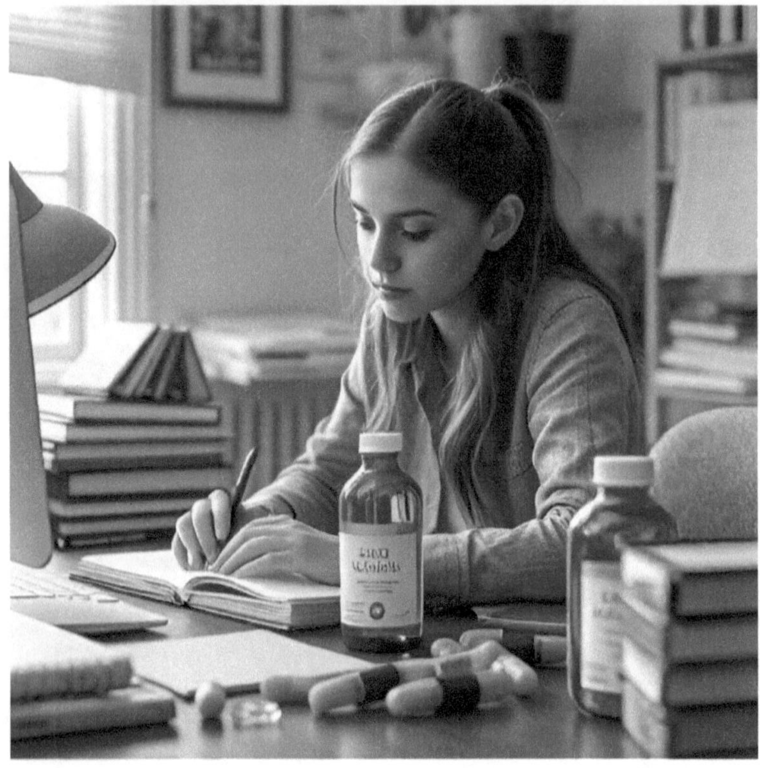

Emily sat at her desk, cluttered with textbooks and half-finished assignments, feeling the familiar pressure of time slipping away. With ADHD, her mind often wandered, flitting from one thought to another like a restless butterfly. Today, however, something felt different; she was determined to confront her focus issues head-on.

After weeks of researching natural remedies and supplements, Emily found herself buried in a sea of information. Each article promised miraculous results—enhanced focus, improved memory, and sustained energy. But as she sorted through the claims, she began to feel overwhelmed. Could something as simple as a supplement really make a difference? Or was she chasing a fantasy in her pursuit of academic success?

Her eyes landed on a bottle of fish oil, highly recommended for its Omega-3 fatty acids, crucial for brain health. Emily remembered her favorite teacher mentioning that these nutrients could help not just with focus but also with emotional regulation. But the leap from hope to trust always felt treacherous; how could she know what would actually work for her?

Determined to find a pathway through her cognitive haze, she decided to try the supplements, integrating them into her daily routine. The first few days yielded minimal changes; her attention still wavered during lectures, and concentration remained elusive during study sessions. Yet, she held onto the glimmer of hope that persistence would yield results.

As weeks turned into a month, Emily noticed subtle shifts. Mornings felt sharper; she was able to maintain focus during her classes longer than ever before. An unfamiliar buoyancy filled her, igniting a fire of enthusiasm she had almost forgotten. Each small victory became a testament to the positive changes taking root within her.

But as with any journey, toward progress often comes the darkness of doubt. Anxiety crept in, whispering fears of regression. What if the supplements were just a temporary fix? What if, deep down, she still struggled with her ADHD, unable to keep up with her peers? Panic clawed at her chest as she approached midterms, a storm of uncertainty brewing in her mind.

On the night before her first exam, with her stomach twisted in knots, Emily found herself second-guessing her choices. Surrounded by the comfort of friends who had chosen different academic paths, who thrived without her struggles, she felt isolated amidst her insecurities. She thought of retreating, giving in to the weight of her challenges instead of stepping boldly into the light.

But just as despair threatened to swallow her whole, she recalled the progress she had made. The supplements had not only offered clarity but also a sense of control she had long craved. As she took a deep breath, steadying her heartbeat, determination flooded back. This moment was not the end; it was an opportunity to harness her experiences and step forward into the unknown.

As Emily penned her final thoughts in her journal, the weight of expectation began to lift. She resolved to embrace her journey with all its jagged edges and unpredictable turns. Tomorrow, she would confront her exam, fortified not just by supplements but by the resilient spirit she had cultivated in the face of adversity.

The Science Behind the Supplements

Research and Studies

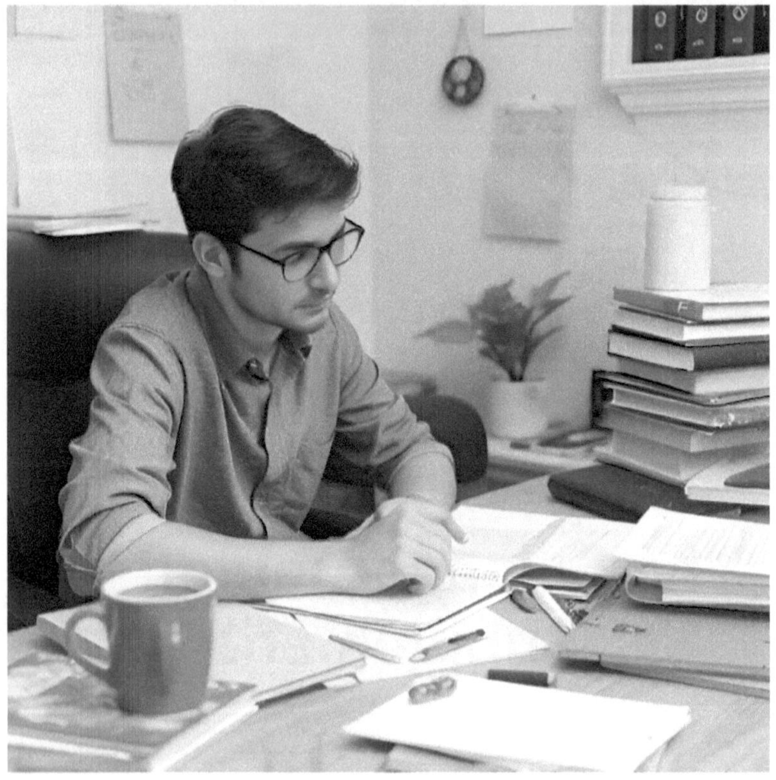

Nathan sat at his cluttered desk, a cup of cold coffee lingering beside his unopened textbooks. The frantic notes scattered around him whispered stories of relentless research, late nights, and early mornings. Driven by an insatiable thirst for knowledge about cognitive supplements, he dived deep into the scholarly articles that framed the landscape of cognitive enhancement. Each study was a piece of an intricate puzzle, revealing the potential benefits and risks of the very substances he had begun incorporating into his daily life.

As he plowed through the findings, Nathan discovered a plethora of studies exhaustedly dissecting various supplements like Omega-3 fatty acids and Ginkgo

Biloba. He noted the consistent references to the enhancement of memory function and improved focus levels that seemed almost too good to be true. With every study he read, he felt a growing sense of obligation to dissect and analyze these claims further. Were they robust enough to build a foundation for his burgeoning regimen? Or were they simply mirages on the horizon of cognitive enhancement?

By the time twilight cast shadows around his dimly lit room, Nathan found himself entangled in a web of conflicting opinions and alarmingly thin evidence. Skepticism clawed at his resolve when he stumbled upon a contrasting study that condemned certain popular supplements, branding them ineffective and, at times, potentially harmful. A wave of anxiety washed over him. Had he placed his trust in a hypothesis that could leave him more vulnerable than before? He could feel the tension building within him, like a coiled spring ready to snap, as the weight of doubt began to overshadow the flickering light of hope he had carried into this research journey.

Debunking Myths

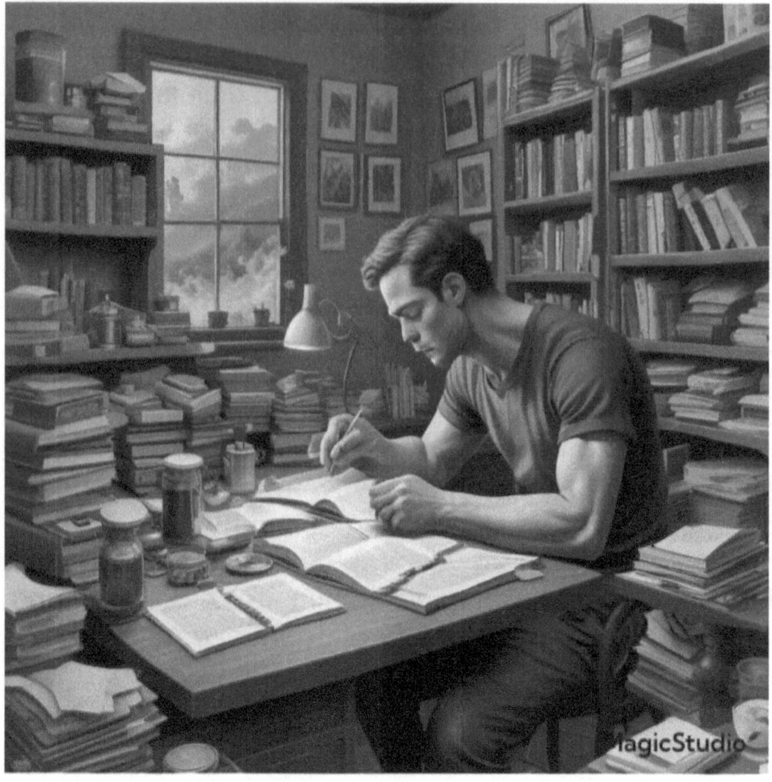

In a world overflowing with information, the realm of cognitive supplements is riddled with misconceptions. Leo, an insightful researcher, finds himself immersed in a complex landscape where anecdotal evidence often overshadows scientific facts. As he delves deeper, he uncovers a myriad of myths—some benign, others dangerously misleading. There's the myth that all supplements are safe simply because they are 'natural'. Unbeknownst to many, the term 'natural' can mask a multitude of potential risks. Skepticism creeps in, and he feels compelled to expose the truth behind these alluring claims.

An alarming myth suggests that consuming large quantities of supplements guarantees superior cognitive function. Leo grimaces as he recalls a friend who bombarded his system with every pill available, convinced it would unlock his brain's full potential. In reality, the body requires balance; too much of a good thing can spiral into adverse effects. With knowledge comes responsibility, and Leo's quest now ignites a fire within him to champion a more educated approach to supplementation.

As he researches, Leo uncovers startling statistics: many cognitive enhancements attributed to supplements are often exaggerated, fueled by marketing ploys rather than scientific proof. Each revelation heightens his urgency; he knows he must share these insights. With a heart full of empathy for those seeking genuine improvement, he prepares for a pivotal discussion with his peers. What if his words reveal uncomfortable truths? What if he disrupts their preconceived notions? The tension swells within him as he steps towards the stage, his voice wavering yet resolute. The quest for cognitive clarity has unleashed a deeper battle against misinformation, and he stands on the brink of a transformative moment.

Emerging Trends in Cognitive Support

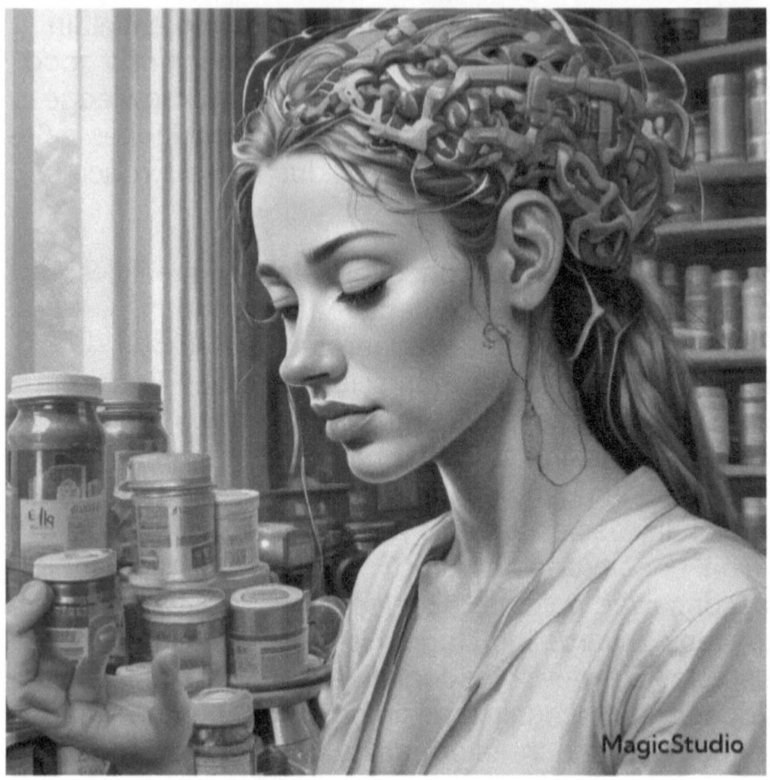

Olivia immersed herself in the latest research, her brow furrowed with concentration. Here she was, on the brink of answering some of the most pressing questions surrounding cognitive support supplements. What innovations awaited on the horizon? What breakthroughs would redefine how individuals approached their cognitive health?

With a surge of excitement, she delved into the world of nootropics, discussing their potential alongside her peers. These cognitive enhancers had captivated the scientific community, showcasing promise not only in boosting memory but also in enhancing focus, creativity, and even emotional resilience. As Olivia spoke, her colleagues nodded, intrigued by the prospects.

Yet, amidst these discussions lay an underlying tension. With every new discovery, skeptics emerged, raising questions about the safety and efficacy of such supplements. Was the market ready to embrace these innovative approaches to cognitive health, or would regulation and public opinion hold back the tide of progress?

Olivia felt the weight of responsibility. She must find a way to bridge the gap between innovation and caution. How could she ensure that those eager to improve their cognitive capabilities were armed with accurate information? With each passing day, the urgency grew. The clock was ticking, and the race to harness these emerging trends had just begun. How many lives could be transformed if she succeeded?

As she gathered her thoughts, the specter of self-doubt lingered. What if society wasn't ready? What if her research led to more questions than answers? Just as these fears began to take hold, a breakthrough appeared on her screen, illuminating the possibilities that lay ahead. Olivia knew she stood at the threshold of something monumental, a pivotal moment that could not only change her life but the lives of countless others seeking a clearer mind and a brighter future. The challenge was now hers to navigate.

The Power of Community

Finding Support Groups

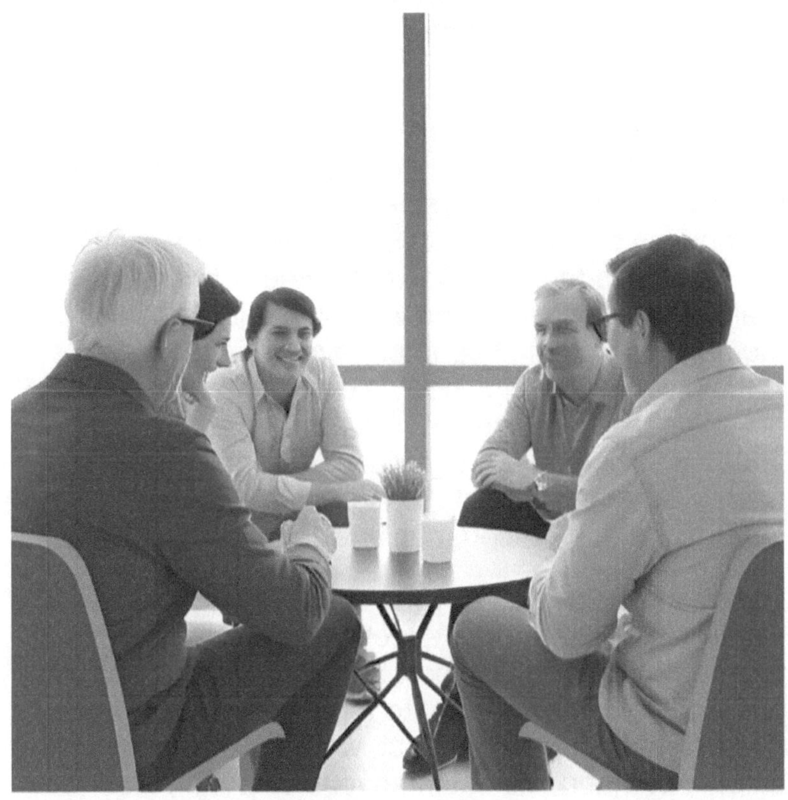

Daniel had always been a solitary figure, navigating the stormy seas of cognitive challenges alone. It wasn't until an old friend mentioned the importance of community that he began to understand the transformative power of connection. With a sense of trepidation, he decided to reach out, searching for local support groups, hoping to find others who were experiencing similar struggles in their cognitive journeys.

His first meeting was a revelation. Seated in a modest room with a circle of earnest faces, each with their own story, Daniel felt an overwhelming sense of belonging. They shared their victories and setbacks, laughter and tears, each sharing strategies that worked and those that failed. The stories intertwined, forming a tapestry of resilience and hope. It wasn't just about cognitive enhancement; it was about lives being transformed, together.

As the meetings continued, Daniel discovered a profound strength within himself. With each session, he was building relationships, learning from others, and sharing his own experiences. However, an unsettling feeling began to creep in. As the weeks passed, Daniel realized that while support was plentiful, one particular member had been absent for several meetings. Curiosity mixed with concern compelled Daniel to reach out. What he found sent a chill down his spine: the absence was due to a significant decline in cognitive health. Suddenly, the stakes felt real, and the importance of their community was magnified tenfold.

Determined not to let anyone slip away unnoticed, Daniel rallied the group, encouraging them to come together not just for support but to actively check on one another. They agreed to form smaller sub-groups and establish regular contact, weaving a stronger safety net that could catch anyone who stumbled.

Yet, as they implemented this new plan, whispers of doubt began to surface. What if they couldn't help everyone? The fear of losing someone to the darkness of cognitive decline lurked just beneath the surface. With it came the realization that every shared story had the potential to reveal painful truths about vulnerability and the fragility of the mind. Their mission now felt heavier, steeped in urgency and the unrelenting question of whether they could be enough.

As Daniel prepared for the next meeting, he couldn't shake the feeling that this was just the beginning of something larger, more demanding. The group had become more than just a source of support; it was now a lifeline, teetering on the brink of both hope and despair. Little did they know that a storm was brewing, one that would test the very fabric of their newfound community.

Online Resources and Forums

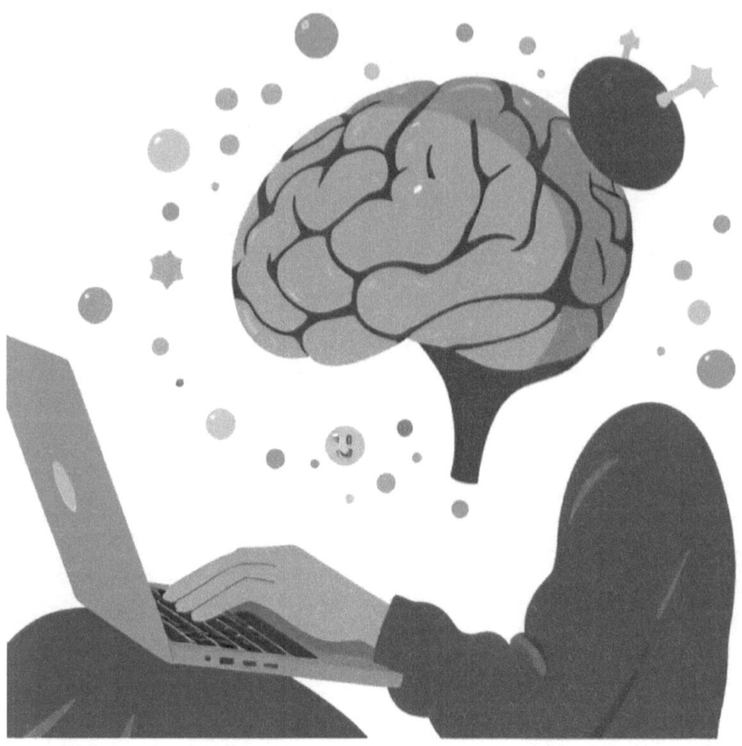

Grace found herself increasingly captivated by the vast array of online resources dedicated to cognitive health. Each click on her laptop unveiled a new world of information, from academic articles to personal blogs recounting individual journeys towards better mental performance. As she delved deeper, she joined forums where people from every walk of life shared their strategies, challenges, and successes in enhancing cognitive health. The sense of a digital community enveloped her—people who understood the struggles she faced.

She began actively participating, sharing her thoughts and engaging in discussions about strategies that worked for others. Secrets shared in the threads felt like intimate conversations, confiding little-known tips about specific supplements and lifestyle changes that could potentially yield impressive results. The forums brimmed with anecdotes that sparked hope and curiosity, and as Grace read stories of transformations, she felt a stirring determination grow within her.

But one day, while scrolling through a thread that offered advice on the latest cognitive supplements, she stumbled upon a post that changed everything. It spoke of a new, untested supplement that had purportedly led to miraculous improvements. As she read the experiences of people claiming exceptional benefits, a flicker of doubt began to creep in. Were these testimonials genuine, or crafted by enthusiasm gone unchecked? Caution battled curiosity, and doubt began to sprinkle its shadows across Grace's initial excitement.

The clock ticked loudly in her room as Grace found herself paralyzed by the decision—should she jump on this new trend, or stick to her trusted routines? The community buzzed with anticipation, spurring her on, yet a quiet voice whispered reminders of sound judgment. Could this be the turning point she needed, or would it derail her progress? Each minute felt heavier, and she felt a collective breath held by an unseen audience, waiting for her next move.

Sharing Success Stories

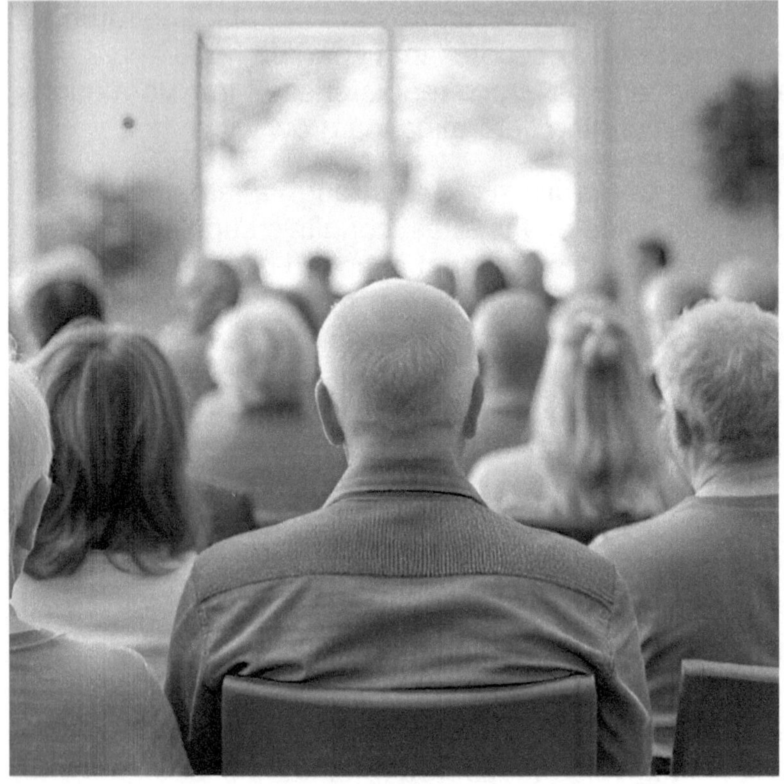

Mark had never imagined that sharing his journey would become a beacon of hope for others. As he settled into his chair at the community center, surrounded by faces of varying ages and backgrounds, he felt a mix of nervousness and excitement. Each person in the room was there for a reason, seeking the same thing he once yearned for—a path to cognitive wellness.

His transformation had begun several months prior, fueled by a desire to sharpen his memory after noticing that simple tasks took longer than before. With a few carefully chosen supplements and a commitment to a healthier lifestyle, Mark had finally settled into a routine that produced results beyond his expectations. As he began to share his story, he could see the glimmers of recognition as others nodded, recalling their own struggles and victories.

Yet, Mark knew that not everyone's journey would mirror his own. Sitting among doctors, students, and working professionals, he felt the weight of their differing aspirations resting heavily on his shoulders. Would his success ignite the same spark in them that had driven him? Or would it only serve as a reminder of their struggles? As he shared his strategies and the personal anecdotes that had colored his experience, he noticed a change in the room—the tension rising as vulnerability cracked through the surface, fearlessly weaving through his narrative.

Mark recounted a particularly challenging day when he nearly gave up, desperately seeking solace and clarity. As he spoke, he could see a reflection of himself in some of their eyes—embarked on a quest fraught with challenges but enriched by community. He urged them to embrace one another's stories as fuel, revealing how communal ties strengthened the very resolve to progress. The room grew warmer with shared understanding, but a mounting sense of urgency pulsated within him. How could he prepare them for setbacks that were sure to come? He wanted to reassure them that during those dark moments, they shouldn't feel alone. They were knitting a tapestry of resilience, stitched together by their experiences.

As he wrapped up his speech, he felt a swell of hope, but a lingering doubt clung closely to his thoughts. Were they truly ready to confront the challenges ahead? Would his words, filled with empathy, be enough to guide them when the road became steep? Just as he was about to leave the center, sharing laughter and exchanging contact information with some of the attendees, he caught a glimpse of a newcomer at the back of the room, a young woman whose expression seemed a blend of hope and despair. Their eyes met briefly, and Mark felt a surge of compulsion igniting within him. He knew his story was not just his own anymore; it belonged to all of them and needed to be shared once again, with renewed vigor and compassion resonating with the pulse of their collective journey.

Culmination of Wisdom

Creating Your Personalized Plan

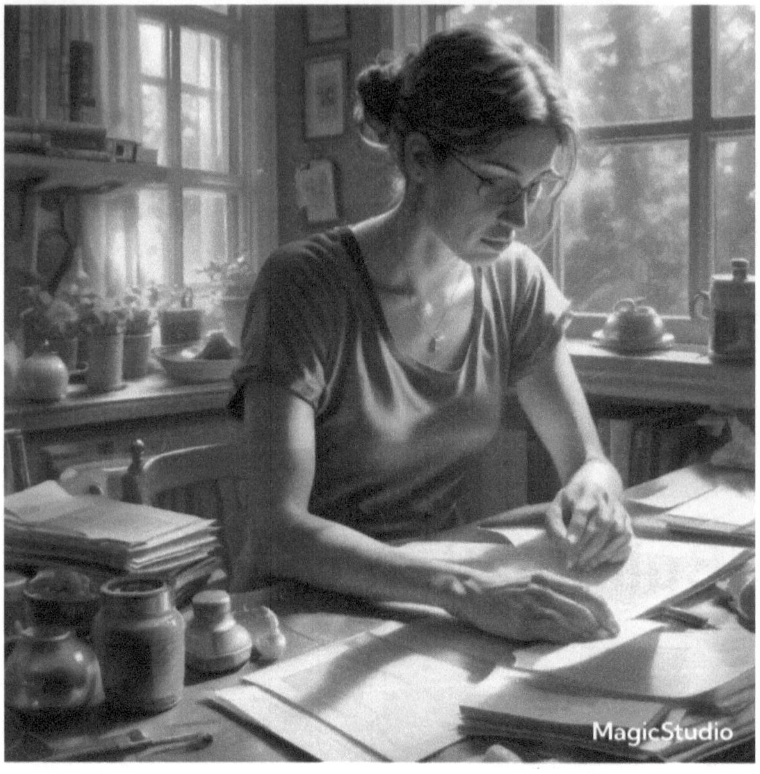

Emily sat at her kitchen table, the sun streaming through the windows, bathing her in a warm glow as she stared at the cluttered mess of papers before her. Notes on cognitive health, tips from friends, and pages torn from health magazines filled the space. This was it—the moment she would finally craft her personalized plan, one that could potentially change her life for the better. Yet, panic surged through her veins. What if she failed yet again?

She took a deep breath, feeling the air fill her lungs, grounding her in the moment. Throughout her journey, Emily learned the significance of taking small steps. Every successful action, no matter how minor, could lead to powerful transformations over time. Yet, she struggled to reconcile this with the enormity of the task ahead. It felt overwhelming, like trying to climb a mountain with no clear path. But she couldn't let fear dictate her journey. She had to believe in herself.

With a pen in hand, she started jotting down her goals. Clarity flooded her thoughts as she aimed for specific outcomes—a daily routine that included her supplements, a mindful eating strategy, and exercise tailored to give her both mental and physical strength. The more she wrote, the more empowered she felt. Each bullet point began to represent not just actions, but the promise of progress. However, as she scribbled down her dreams for cognitive health, doubt echoed in the back of her mind, challenging her resolve.

As the day passed, Emily constructed her plan layer by layer, but a nagging voice whispered of the potential pitfalls she could encounter. What if the supplements didn't work? What if she lost motivation? Just then, her phone buzzed—a reminder for a meeting with her mentor. Was she ready to discuss her plan, to lay bare her aspirations and fears? The thought made her stomach twist with anxiety. Would her mentor see her plan as naive, an illusion crafted from desperation?

The evening approached, and Emily reviewed her plan. Every ounce of her being ached with the desire for success—clearly outlined strategies mingled with an overarching fear of failure. But beneath that fear, a flicker of hope ignited. If she could present her plan and articulate her journey, perhaps she could gain the support she desperately needed. Her pulse quickened as she dialed the number, teetering on the edge of uncertainty, not knowing that this moment would catalyze a wave of challenges yet to emerge.

The line connected, and her mentor's familiar voice greeted her, blending warmth with professionalism. As she dove into her plans, Emily could feel the tension mounting—a mixture of eagerness and dread. Would they validate her hard work, or would they poke holes through her carefully constructed vision? With the air thick with anticipation, Emily realized she had nothing to lose but the chains of doubt that had held her back for far too long.

Yet, as she spoke, a sudden shift in her mentor's tone made her heart race. "Emily, while I appreciate your enthusiasm, we need to discuss the challenges you might face. Often, the path isn't as simple as it seems, and..." The words hung ominously in the air, an unspoken warning—what if the hurdles were greater than she could manage? The tension multiplied, and Emily's heart pounded in her chest. The culmination of her wisdom was about to be tested in ways she never imagined.

Staying Informed: Beyond the Basics

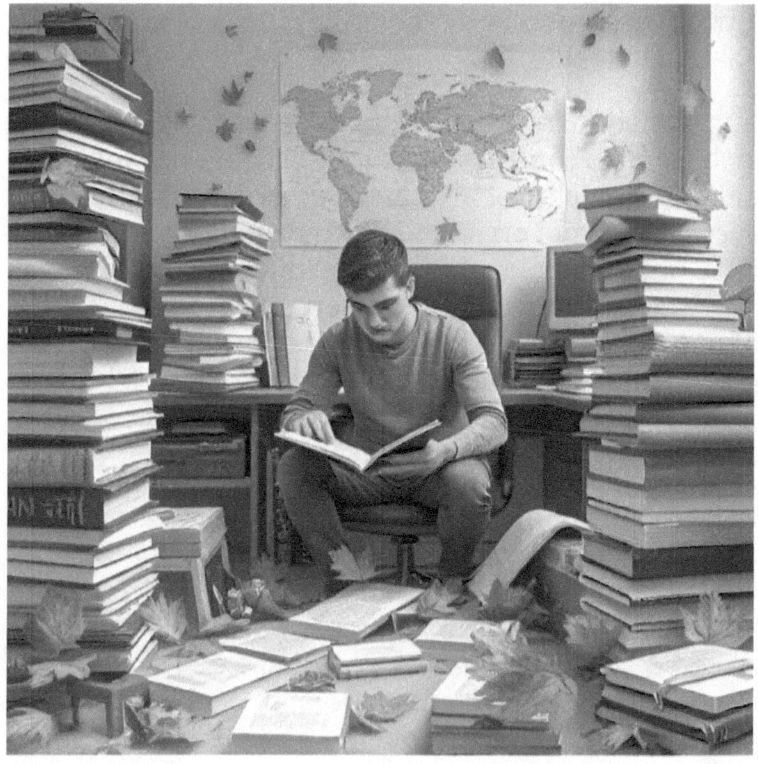

Jordan sat at his cluttered desk, surrounded by stacks of books and articles scattered like fallen leaves in autumn. Each piece of paper contained knowledge that could enhance his cognitive health, yet he felt overwhelmed by the sheer volume of information available. He had learned the fundamental principles of cognitive supplements, but the deeper nuances eluded him. The compelling question nagged at him—how could he stay informed about the latest findings and advancements without drowning in data?

He recalled his last conversation with Emily, who spoke passionately about the importance of lifelong learning. "Staying informed isn't just a choice; it's a commitment," she had said. "The world of cognitive health evolves rapidly, and what worked yesterday might be obsolete tomorrow. We have to stay ahead of the game." This resonated with Jordan more than he realized then, but now, as he stared at the endless possibilities, it felt like a daunting task.

Determined to take action, he began setting aside time each week to read scientific journals, attend webinars, and participate in local health workshops. Each new piece of information added a brushstroke to the canvas of his understanding, but it was not without its challenges. The more he learned, the more he felt the burden of responsibility to keep pace with these advancements. What if he fell behind? What if he missed crucial updates that could benefit his cognitive journey?

As he delved deeper, Jordan uncovered a vibrant community of like-minded individuals dedicated to the pursuit of cognitive health. Online forums buzzed with discussions about recent studies, while local meet-ups offered a space for sharing personal experiences and strategies. It was exhilarating to connect with others on parallel journeys, yet amidst the shared enthusiasm, there were whispers of doubt lurking in his mind. Was he truly equipped to differentiate between credible research and marketing ploys masquerading as science?

He combed through articles, eager to discern fact from fiction. One evening, as he stumbled upon a headline proclaiming a revolutionary supplement that promised to enhance cognitive functions overnight, his heart raced. The claims sounded enticing, yet the skepticism in him rose like a tide. Was this just another fleeting trend? He knew he needed to maintain a critical eye, yet how could he balance skepticism with the hope of genuine advancement?

In the coming weeks, Jordan's tension mounted. He faced a critical decision: to pursue this newly discovered supplement, meticulously researched and recommended by some, or to rely on the trusted methods he had gradually incorporated into his life. The stakes felt higher than ever, as he navigated the waters of cognitive health, fully aware that the wrong choice could set back his progress.

As the day of decision arrived, he could feel the weight of uncertainty pressing on his chest. He questioned whether he would regret not following the crowd or if, by standing firm in his cautious approach, he would avoid potential pitfalls. Inspiration struck him like a jolt—he realized the importance of not only personal growth but of extending his pursuit of knowledge to others. Sharing insights with peers and seeking their perspectives could be the bridge he needed to solidify his understanding.

With his resolve strengthened, he decided to share his findings with Emily and others in the community. Perhaps their collective wisdom could guide him through this fog of uncertainty. As he typed out a message to set up a casual discussion, Jordan felt a flicker of hope. He was not alone in his journey, and together, they could cultivate a culture of informed decision-making that transcended individual pursuit.

The Lifelong Journey of Cognitive Care

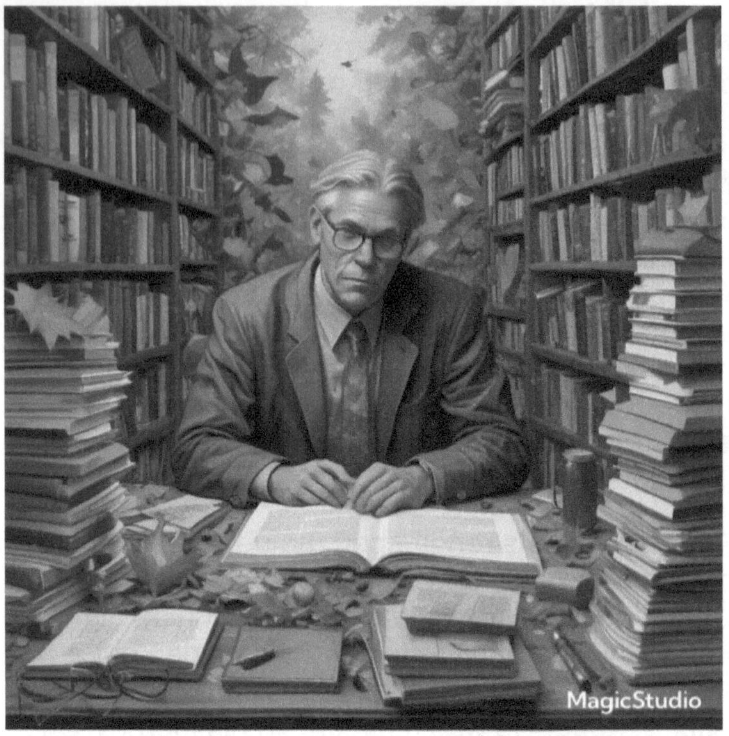

Sam stood at the threshold of a new beginning, the weight of his previous choices swirling in his mind. He thought back to the times he bypassed self-care for fleeting success. As he looked towards the horizon, he knew this path demanded more than mere interest; it required commitment, resilience, and an understanding that cognitive health was a dynamic journey, not a destination.

With each passing week, he implemented changes in his routine, curious about the effects on his mental clarity. He subscribed to podcasts, attended workshops, and surrounded himself with like-minded individuals. The stories of others who had faced cognitive challenges ignited a fire within him, compelling him to delve deeper into practices that supported brain health. Knowledge became his ally as he sought to intertwine science with lifestyle.

But the journey was far from simple. Just when he felt a surge of mastery over his routine, an unexpected setback echoed through his life like the tolling of a bell. Stress from work mounted, resurfacing old habits that enshrouded him in doubt. Each sleepless night turned into prolonged moments of frustration, where instead of clarity, the haze of confusion reigned supreme.

In the thick of this turmoil, Sam leaned on his community. He shared his struggles openly, and in their responses, he found solace. Little did he know, the wisdom hidden in their experiences would propel his journey in unforeseen ways. They reminded him that setbacks were not signs of failure, but integral chapters in the narrative of growth and resilience.

Determined, he identified his triggers, formulating a recovery plan that boasted flexibility combined with structure. Armed with knowledge and a support network, he adjusted his expectations and reassured himself that this was merely a detour—a chance to recalibrate his goals. As the pieces began to align, a sense of empowerment washed over him.

Sam realized that cognitive care was not a sprint, but a marathon—a lifelong engagement with himself, balanced on the knife's edge of ambition and well-being. As he pondered this newfound understanding, the words of his mentor echoed in his mind: Embrace the process, for therein lies the true essence of wisdom. With renewed determination to push through the haze, Sam prepared himself for the adventures yet to unfold in his quest for cognitive mastery.

Facing Setbacks

Understanding Plateaus

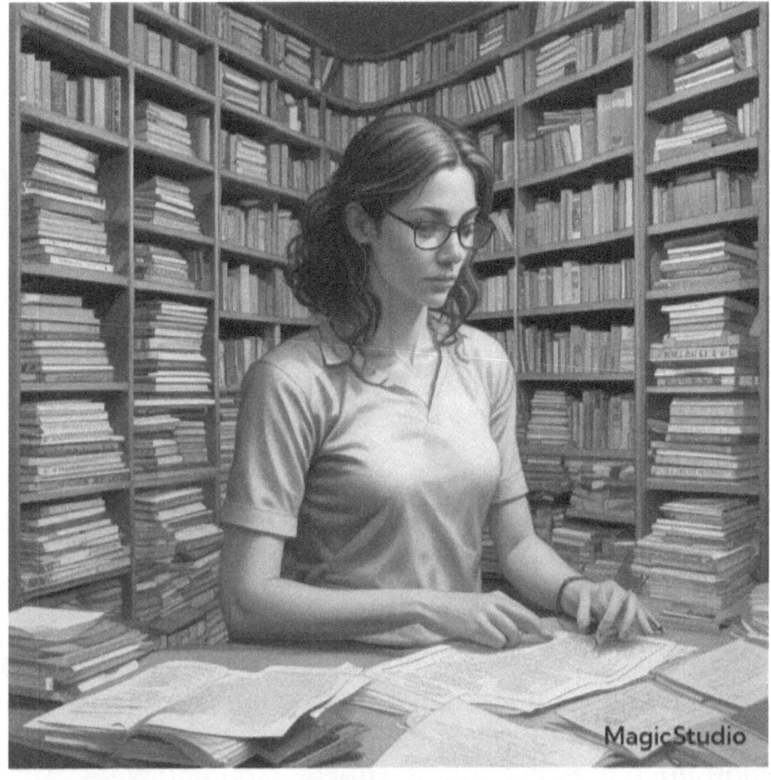

Emma stood in front of her desk, staring at the stacks of notes and the array of colorful highlighters that had once filled her with enthusiasm. Now, they felt like an insurmountable wall. After months of diligent study and unwavering commitment to enhancing her cognitive abilities, she had reached what she could only describe as a plateau. The excitement of rapid progress had faded, replaced by a frustrating stagnation that mirrored her growing anxiety.

She had read about cognitive plateaus, those moments when growth feels stunted despite a rigorous routine. The promise of newfound capabilities that once surged through her veins now felt like a whisper in the wind. Determined to understand this phenomenon, Emma dove deep into research. She learned that plateaus were natural—part of the learning process that even the most successful individuals faced. It was a time for patience, resilience, and strategic adjustment.

But the knowledge did little to soothe her turmoil. As days turned into weeks without visible improvement, the self-doubt began to gnaw at her. What if this is as good as it gets? she thought, the weight of the question pressing heavily on her mind. She sought support from friends, but their encouragement often felt like distant echoes against her inner turmoil. The pressure of her goals loomed larger, each tick of the clock amplifying her desperation.

One evening, in the dim light of her cramped apartment, Emma sat cross-legged on her bedroom floor strewn with papers. She took a deep breath, desperately trying to find a flicker of hope amid the darkness. It was time to navigate her plateau thoughtfully. Armed with journals overflowing with ideas and strategies, she began to map out a plan, knowing that breaking through would require not just renewed effort but a reevaluation of what worked and what didn't.

As she penned down her thoughts, the tension in her heart twisted tighter. Every strategy she listed felt tainted with doubt—what if these plans failed, too? Could she really turn the tide? The room grew quiet, save for the sound of her pen scratching against paper, increasingly frantic as time flowed through her fingers. Emma was acutely aware that soon, she would have to confront the world again—without the certainty she craved, and with everything she held dear hanging in the balance.

Revisiting Your Strategy

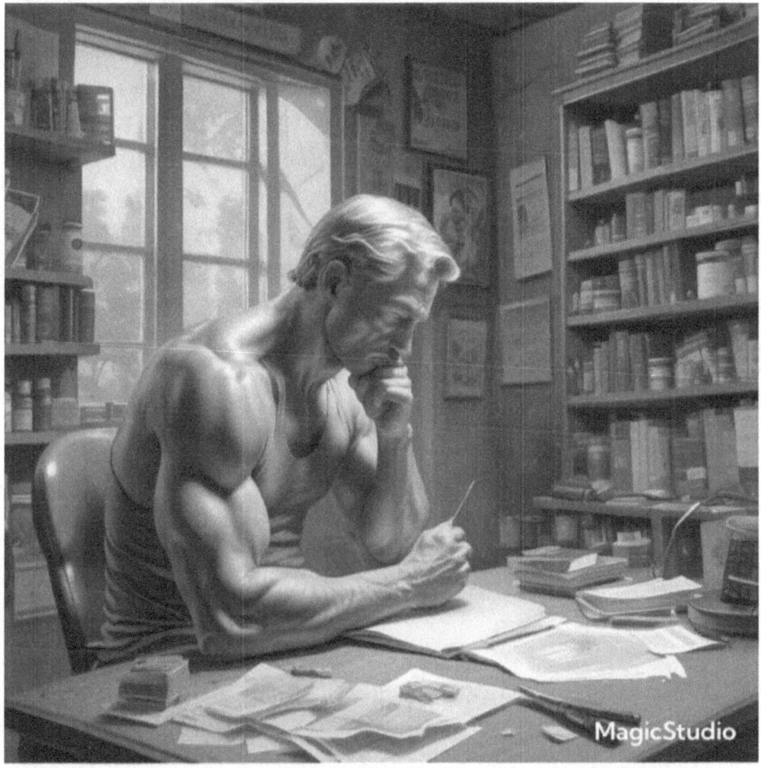

As Mike sat at his desk, the weight of his cognitive journey pressed heavily upon him. Days had turned into weeks, and yet the progress he had anticipated seemed to elude him, fading like a whisper in the wind. In the quiet corners of his mind, doubt began to creep in. Was he really doing enough to improve his cognitive abilities? Was the effort he was putting into his supplements and routine yielding any real results?

He had meticulously crafted a strategy that encompassed everything he had learned: the right supplements, a balanced diet, and mindfulness practices. Yet, despite his tenacity, he felt stuck—adrift in a sea of uncertainty. The challenges he faced were now more than just obstacles; they felt like insurmountable walls blocking his way toward success.

Mike took a deep breath and attempted to refocus, but the frustration began to morph into a gnawing anxiety.

Determined to regain control, Mike decided it was time to revisit his approach. Was he too rigid in his methods? Perhaps he was missing a vital component that could spark the change he desperately sought. With fresh resolve, he dove back into research and reflection, sifting through his notes. Each word he read ignited a flickering hope that perhaps a small adjustment could ignite a powerful transformation.

As he meticulously retraced his steps, reality dawned on him. This detour—this moment of stagnation—was not an end but a vital part of his journey. The trials had taught him resilience, had nudged him to innovate, and had awakened a deeper understanding of his own needs. And so, with renewed clarity, Mike plotted his next steps, aware that even setbacks held the potential for profound growth.

But as he reviewed his notes, plotting various adjustments, he could not shake the feeling of an impending storm. Outside his window, dark clouds gathered ominously, foreshadowing the challenges that lay ahead. Unbeknownst to him, the revisions he was about to make would not only test his strategy but also his spirit.

Learning from Mistakes

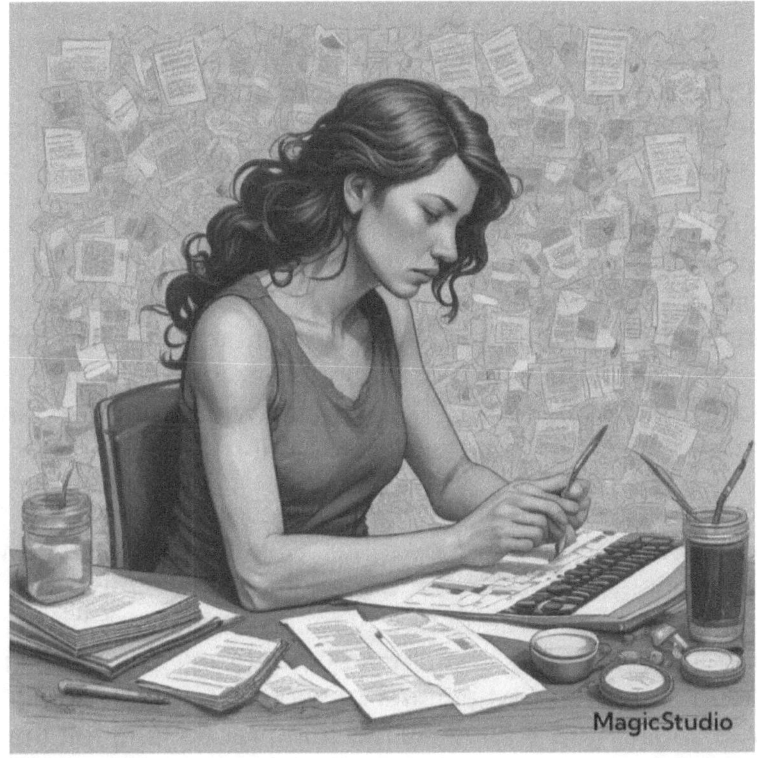

Sophia sat at her desk, surrounded by scattered notes and a half-empty cup of cold coffee. The weight of her recent setbacks loomed heavily over her, a constant reminder of the mistakes she had made in her cognitive health journey. Her attempts to optimize her brain function through various supplements had not yielded the expected results, leaving her frustrated and disheartened.

In moments of quiet reflection, Sophia replayed her missteps: the impulsive decisions to try every new supplement that came her way, the lack of patience when results didn't appear overnight, and the neglect of foundational habits like sleep and nutrition. Each mistake felt like a stone added to the backpack she carried, making her progress feel unbearably slow.

Yet in the depths of her despair, she realized that within those misjudgments lay invaluable lessons. Instead of viewing her setbacks as failures, she began to see them as stepping stones. Each error was an opportunity for growth, a chance to build resilience. Determined to reclaim her journey, Sophia grabbed her journal and began to write.

She listed her mistakes, from disregarding the importance of a balanced diet to underestimating the role of stress management in cognitive health. Next to each, she penned down the insight it brought—like the necessity of a holistic approach rather than relying solely on supplements. The words flowed from her pen, transforming her frustration into clarity.

As she delved deeper into her reflections, a sense of empowerment washed over her. She envisioned a new path: one grounded in understanding, where mistakes were not to be hidden but embraced as intricate parts of her story. But as she closed her journal, an unsettling thought crept in—what if her newfound understanding was challenged again? As her mind raced, she felt the tension build, the uncertainty of what lay ahead pulsating in her chest.

In that moment, Sophia knew she was at a crossroads. Would she let future setbacks define her, or would she rise to face them with the strength of her newfound wisdom? The question echoed in her mind, amplifying her resolve as she prepared to navigate an uncertain road ahead.

The Future of Cognitive Health

Innovations in Supplementation

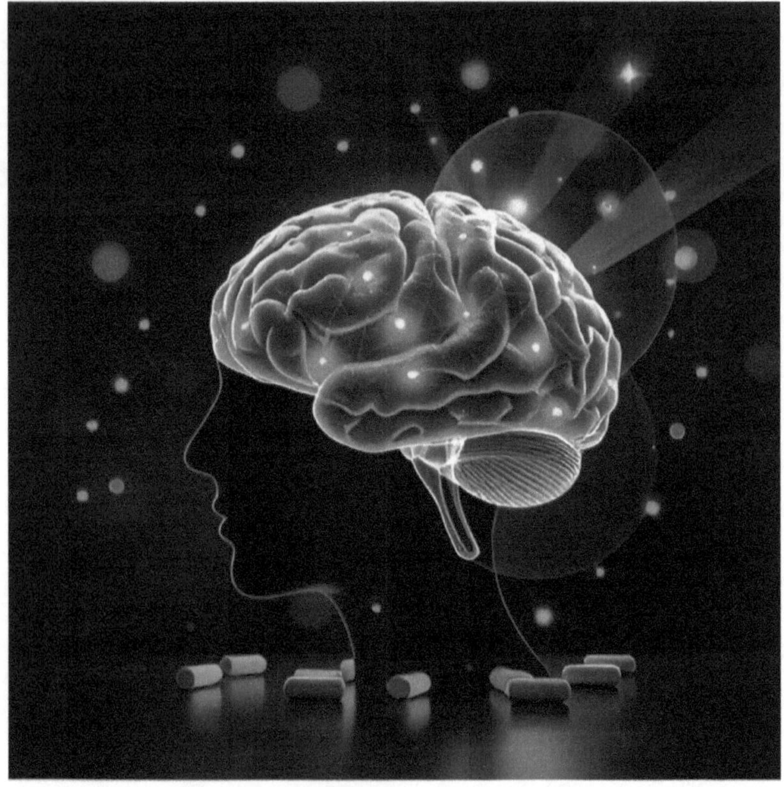

Nathan found himself perched on the edge of his desk, his heart racing with anticipation as he discovered the emerging innovations in cognitive supplementation. With news buzzing about the latest advancements, he couldn't help but marvel at the potential these innovations held to transform cognitive health. It wasn't just scientific jargon to him; it was a promise, a beacon of hope for professionals and students alike hopelessly braving the struggles of mental fatigue and focus.

As he dug deeper, Nathan uncovered cutting-edge nootropic compounds gaining traction in research circles. These weren't mere supplements; they were meticulously crafted blends that promised to enhance cognitive function dramatically. He read about the trials conducted by leading neuroscientists, showcasing remarkable improvements in attention, memory recall, and even emotional regulation. Each study fueled his resolve to explore these advancements further, believing that they might offer him the edge he desperately sought.

However, amid the excitement lay a lingering caution. Nathan felt a pang of anxiety as he overheard a conversation in an online forum, where skeptics dismissed these new developments as mere fads or dangerous hype. The tension rippled through the community, as questions about safety, efficacy, and ethical implications surfaced. Would these innovations genuinely pave the way for improved cognitive health, or were they built on the shaky foundation of exploitation and hope? The prospect both thrilled and unnerved him, driving Nathan to the precipice of a decision that could change the trajectory of his cognitive health journey.

As the clock ticked, a thought crossed Nathan's mind, darkening the atmosphere. What if the answers he sought remained just out of reach? What if, in a quest for better mental clarity, he inadvertently wandered into treacherous territory where the line between science and marketing blurred? He could feel the weight of uncertainty pressing down on him, urging him to act, to choose—yet fearful of taking a misstep.

The Role of Technology

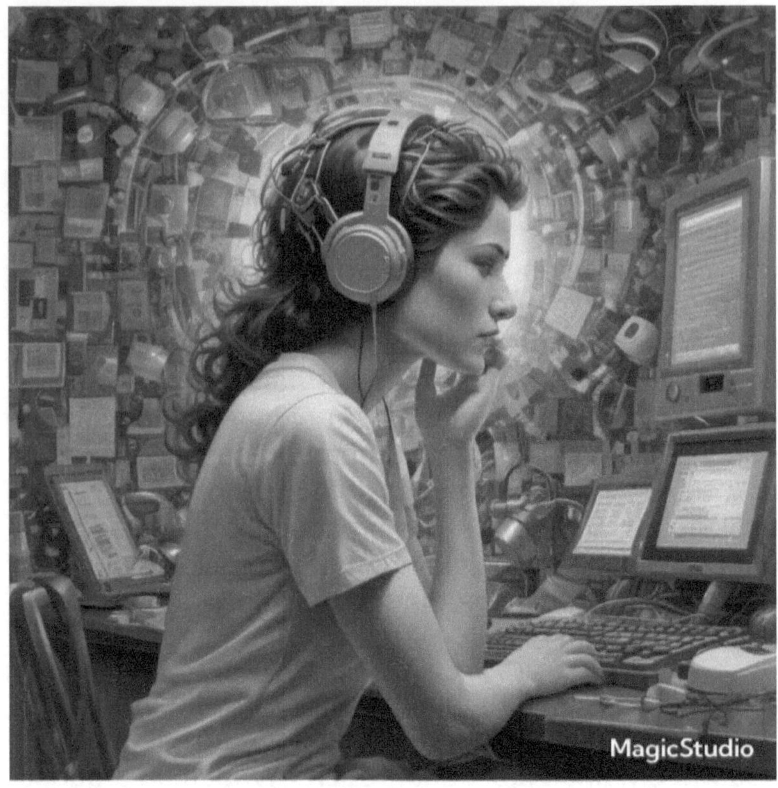

Julia often found herself lost in the chaos of her digital life, with notifications pinging relentlessly and distractions vying for her attention. However, amid this noise, she also recognized that technology could be a powerful ally in her journey towards cognitive wellness. Embracing the right tools could transform the way she approached her mental health and academic success.

With a surge of determination, she explored an array of cognitive-enhancing applications tailored to improve focus, mindfulness, and memory. Guided by user reviews and expert recommendations, she selected a few that promised to align with her goals. The first was a meditation app that offered guided sessions specifically designed for students under stress. As she began to weave these sessions into her routine, she felt an unexpected calm wash over her, sharpening her ability to concentrate.

Equipped with her smartphone, Julia downloaded a brain-training game that claimed to boost cognitive function through engaging challenges and puzzles. Each evening, she dedicated time to play, enjoying not only the challenge but also the tangible improvements in her critical thinking skills. She started noticing that tasks—once daunting and overwhelming—became more manageable with her newfound clarity.

However, amidst her digital journey, she faced unexpected moments of doubt. Late one night, while catching up on her studies, she became overwhelmed by the competing demands of her coursework and the seductive ease of social media. As she scrolled through images of success and happiness, her heart sank. Despite her best efforts, she felt a creeping sense of inadequacy gnawing at her confidence. Julia began to question whether technology was truly her ally or simply another layer of distraction.

Just when the tension felt insurmountable, she stumbled upon a community forum dedicated to cognitive health and technology. Here, she found stories of fellow students grappling with the same internal struggles, confronting their digital dependencies. Slowly, a sense of hope blossomed within her, reigniting her commitment to use technology not to escape reality but to embrace it, transforming her tools into instruments of empowerment rather than hindrance.

As she navigated this delicate balance, Julia felt a compelling urge to share her journey. She began writing blog posts, detailing her experiences with different apps, tips for setting boundaries with technology, and her progress toward cognitive health.

The response was overwhelming—fellow students flooded her inbox with gratitude and shared their stories of overcoming their own challenges. Not only was Julia rallying a community, but she was also solidifying her own path forward.

Yet, just as she felt a surge of momentum, the pressure mounted. With exams around the corner, her reliance on technology intensified, leading her back to moments of doubt. What had started as a supportive tool now felt like an additional weight on her shoulders. Would she succumb to the noise again? As the clock ticked down to her first exam, she pondered whether she could truly harness technology to bolster her cognitive health, fearing one last step might tip her balance entirely.

Looking Ahead: What Science Says

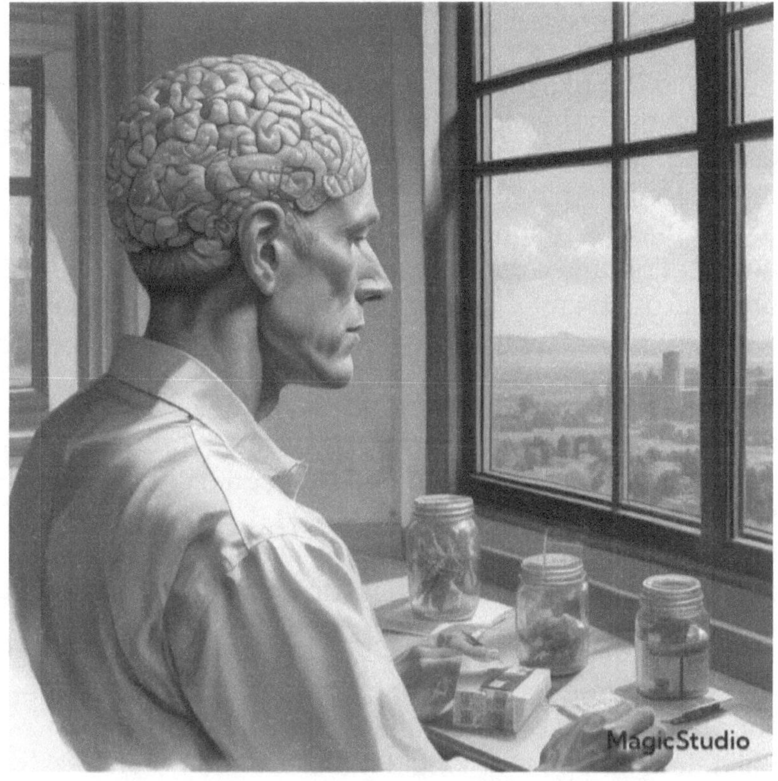

As Leo gazed out of the window, his mind race with thoughts of the future. The advancements in cognitive health research had been remarkable, but what lay just over the horizon was where the true curiosity sparked. He recalled the recent discussions he'd had with his peers at the university—a group of passionate researchers committed to pushing the boundaries of what was known about cognitive enhancement.

One particular study focused on neuroplasticity had thrilled him; it suggested that the brain could rewire itself more efficiently than previously thought. Leo pondered the implications. If they could harness this understanding and develop therapies that could aid in rejuvenation of cognitive faculties, what would that mean for professionals burning out in bustling careers? What about students struggling under the weight of countless responsibilities?

But amid the excitement, a murmur of doubt lingered. Science did not yield its secrets easily. The trials were grueling, fraught with questions that could derail the most promising theories. As Leo flipped through pages of complex data sheets, his heart raced with both anticipation and apprehension. What if the breakthroughs they envisioned faltered? What if they were led astray by their own ambitions?

Suddenly, a notification pinged on his desktop. An upcoming symposium on cognitive health promised to unveil groundbreaking findings that could change the landscape of cognitive supplements. Leo felt a surge of determination; he would be there, and he would gather every piece of information available. This was not just another day—it was a turning point.

As he prepared for the event, Leo could not shake the lingering feeling of uncertainty. Would the research validate his hopes, or would it expose the harsh realities of limitations? In the shadows of innovation lay the potential for disappointment, and as he sat surrounded by his notes, he realized his journey was about more than just knowledge. It was about the voices, the stories of people longing for relief from cognitive fatigue, and they deserved answers.

Days later, under the blinding lights of the conference hall, anticipation buzzed like electricity in the air. Researchers spoke passionately about their findings, illustrating the delicate dance between neurons that could lead to enhanced cognitive function. Leo scribbled furiously, eager to catch every fragment of insight. Yet, as the final speaker approached the podium, tension gripped him. Could the final piece of this puzzle hold the revelation everyone had been waiting for? Or would it evanesce into the realm of speculative science?

The room fell silent. He held his breath, awaiting the conclusions that could reshape not only academic theories but also the everyday lives of countless individuals. Leo was acutely aware that what came next could illuminate a brighter path forward—or cast doubt into the minds of those yearning for progress. As the words echoed in his ears, he understood this was not just a breakthrough; this was the front line of a revolution waiting to unfurl its wings.

Acknowledgement

I extend my heartfelt appreciation to my husband for his unwavering support and selfless dedication throughout the creation of this book. His tireless efforts behind the scenes have been instrumental in shaping this material into a work that I hope will be both enriching and worthwhile for our readers. His encouragement, patience, and invaluable insights have truly made a difference, and I am deeply grateful for his partnership in this endeavor.

About The Author

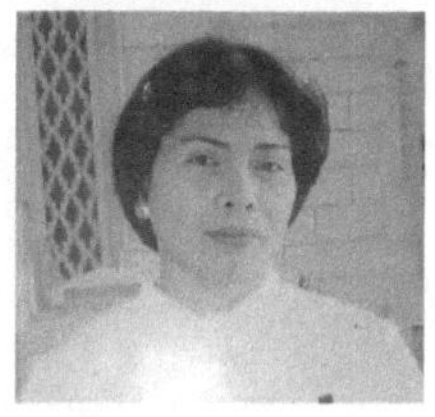

Nena Buenaventura is a dedicated leader with a rich and diverse career spanning healthcare and business. Her unwavering commitment to service first manifested in healthcare, where she spearheaded departments, empowering patients to reclaim their health and independence. Driven by an entrepreneurial spirit, she transitioned to the business world, deepening her understanding of finance and entrepreneurship. Nena's multifaceted journey culminates in her prolific writing, where she shares her knowledge and insights across a range of disciplines, connecting with readers on a personal and intellectual level.

 Through her impactful work in healthcare, business, and writing, Nena continues to make a lasting difference in the world.

Books List Authored by Nena Buenaventura

https://www.amazon.com/s?k=nena+buenaventura&crid=ZPXJQTNTWN13&qid=1730469536&sprefix=nena+buenaventura+the+art+of+living%2Caps%2C457&ref=sr_pg_1

www.ingramcontent.com/pod-product-compliance
Lightning Source LLC
Chambersburg PA
CBHW021147260726
48656CB00025B/1611